Erectile Dysfunction and Prostate Problems

By Li Zheng and Changhong Zhou

Edited by Steven Zhou

Dedicated to my family and patients who give me the
motivation to help people become happier and healthier

Acknowledgements

I would like to thank my daughter who is willing to find time to help me edit my book while she could have spent time with her friends. I greatly admire her passion for the nature and knowledge, and she has taught me how to access the newest scientific knowledge. She always gives me background knowledge to help me understand why young women and men in modern society have certain kinds of unhealthy behaviors, and she makes me connect my professional knowledge with modern life experiences, which I would have never understood because I grew up in a completely different environment.

I would like to thank my parents who had worked hard their whole lives. I learned from them that knowledge, rather than money, can help me lead a fulfilling life. I learned from their disciplined lifestyles to enjoy all the happiness my work has brought me. Their lifelong experiences taught me that if you do not dedicate yourself to taking care of yourself, nobody else can help you achieve a happier and healthier life.

I would also like to thank my husband, who dedicates much of his time and energy to scientific research without thinking about money or a life of luxury. He helps me take care of my three kids and provided me with the time and opportunity to write this book.

Li Zheng

Foreword

Dr. Li Zheng and her husband, Dr. Changhong Zhou, have had many years of a very successful clinical practice in acupuncture and Chinese herbal medicine. This publication continues Dr. Zheng's series of books describing details of how acupuncture and Chinese herbs have provided health benefits for many patients that have come to her for treatment over the years. The focus of this book is on male sexual function issues, specifically erectile dysfunction and enlargement of the prostate gland, which are very common health problems for older men. The presentation includes especially case studies, which make the book easily readable and interesting. Dr. Zheng's writing follows individual patients over the courses of their histories with her clinic. The style is very straightforward, including difficulties encountered along the way as well as successes. This book should be of interest, not only for men looking for effective treatments for erectile dysfunction or prostate enlargement, but also for healthcare practitioners who want to gain more insight about acupuncture and Chinese herbal medicine.

Donald Godfrey, Professor Emeritus
Department of Neurology and Division of Otolaryngology and Dentistry, Department of Surgery, University of Toledo

Contents

Part I ED and Low Testosterone

Part II Prostate Problems and Elevated PSA

Introduction

It has become increasingly common for young men to develop prostate problems and erectile dysfunction (ED) in their forties or even in their late thirties. However, most of the common treatments for prostate problems provide only temporary fixes. For example, while surgery can remove out part of or the entire prostate to relieve pressure on the bladder, men tend to experience impotence and urine incontinence post-op. Similarly, treatments such as testosterone pills and injections may initially increase testosterone levels and sex drive, but overtime men will gradually lose their ability to produce their testosterone naturally due to artificial supplementation. Furthermore, the use of artificial testosterone carries a plethora of negative side effects, including high blood pressure, increased sweating and body odor, and accelerated prostate enlargement.

In my research, I followed many patients for over ten years after they began testosterone injections shortly after undergoing prostate surgery. Unfortunately, the symptoms returned within a few years following the treatment. If the underlying causes of elevated PSA level, frequent urination, and rapid testosterone levels drops were not addressed, the effectiveness of the medication would diminish. Consequently, they had to increase the dosage of the medication, leading to additional side effect such as insomnia.

With twenty-seven years of clinical experience, I have discovered the most common root causes of ED and prostate enlargement. Combining Acupuncture and Chinese herbs to treat patients with ED and elevated PSA levels, I have observed that individuals who make early lifestyle and dietary changes achieve the best therapeutic effects. As they adjust their habits, their testosterone levels gradually increase, leading to stronger and reduced urgency to urinate. By making lifestyle modifications they can minimize their reliance on medication using the lowest possible dosage with fewer side effects. In this book, I present clinical case studies and scientific research to emphasize the crucial role of lifestyle choices in maintaining long-term health and happiness for young men, even into their seventies or eighties. Regulating alcohol consumption, adapting a nutritious diet, engaging in regular exercise, and a strong relationship with their partner, are all essential factors.

By combining herbal medicine with regular acupuncture treatments, even seventy-year-old men can experience restful sleep, sexual activity and an enjoyable life with their partners. Conversely, men who solely rely on surgery and medications without a willing to change their lifestyle face a higher risk of losing their sexual function in their early fifties. Additionally, they may frequently worry about simple task such as finding the nearest restroom and experiencing memory loss at the peak of their careers. Those who are stubborn-minded will become frustrated when they realize that their energy level, memory, and sex drive are even lower than those of some men who are eighty years old.

While it is true that some individuals with erectile dysfunction can still lead fulfilling lives into old age, it is crucial to strive for stronger muscles, normal hormone levels, and sharp memory. Although perfection cannot be guaranteed, we can make efforts to improve our well-being, allowing us to live vibrant and fulfilling lives regardless of age.

Part I

ED and Low Testosterone

Chapter 1

Low Testosterone and Impotence

Testosterone, a steroid hormone produced by the interstitial cells of the testes, plays a crucial role. The production of testosterone is controlled by a luteinizing hormone released by the anterior pituitary gland and is subject to a negative feedback mechanism. This means that if you have too much testosterone, the pituitary gland will reduce the release of luteinizing hormone so that the testes produce less testosterone. On the other hand, if testosterone level is too low, the pituitary will produce more of the stimulating hormone to push the testes to produce more testosterone.

The functions of testosterone:

1. Testosterone is needed for the proper development of the male reproductive system during puberty.

2. Following puberty, testosterone keeps the male reproductive system working properly and producing healthy sperm and seminal fluid.

3. Testosterone promotes sexual function and sexual drive.

4. Testosterone initiates and maintains the secondary sex characteristics of males. Males exhibit increased muscular

development, deepened voice, broad shoulders, body and facial hair, and patterned baldness.

What can cause low testosterone level and erectile dysfunction?

Stress:

Research indicates that stress can lower testosterone levels temporarily, causing functional impotence. But if stress continues for too long, structural changes will follow.

Medications:

Certain medications, such as the drugs for high blood pressure, anti-anxiety, antidepressants (including the tricyclics and the monoamine oxidase inhibitors) and narcotics, have been implicated in erectile dysfunction, decreased sexual drive, decreased libido, and impaired ejaculation. Most high blood pressure medications have been associated with some erectile impairment, but diuretics seem to have little effect on erectile function. Calcium channel blockers and acetylcholine esterase inhibitors are associated with a low incidence of erectile dysfunction. High blood pressure medications that target the sympathetic nervous system seldom cause impotence but can cause retrograde ejaculation because of the relaxation of the smooth muscles in the prostatic urethra and bladder neck.

Thus, if one kind of blood pressure pill causes temporary impotence, you should try another kind.

Generally, erectile dysfunction due to taking selective serotonin reuptake inhibitors (SSRIs), should resolve itself after discontinuing this medication. In the January 2008 issue of the *Journal of Sexual Medicine*, Dr. Csoka and colleagues in the University of Pittsburgh-Medicine reported three cases of SSRI-related sexual dysfunctions such as low libido, inability to achieve orgasm, loss of sensation in genital area, and erectile dysfunction. All three patients took SSRIs. Their sex function did not return to normal level after they stopped the medication. The first case was a 29-year-old young man. He showed permanent erectile dysfunction after taking fluoxetine 20 mg once daily for a 4-month period. His erectile capacity was temporarily restored with injectable Alprostadil, a medicine that increases blood flow to penis by expanding the blood vessel. The second case was a 44-year-old male. He showed persistent loss of libido, loss of sensation in genital area, ejaculatory anhedonia (inability to experience joy from ejaculation), and erectile dysfunction after taking 20-mg of citalopram once daily for 18 months. His erectile function was restored with oral Viagra, but the other symptoms remained. The third case was a 28-year-old male. He developed similar symptoms after taking several different SSRIs over a 2-year period. His symptoms were improved with extended-release methylphenidate, a central nervous system stimulant. The researchers concluded that SSRIs can cause long-term effects on all aspects of the sexual response cycle that may persist after the drugs were discontinued. They speculated that the mechanism may involve persistent changes in endocrine and epigenetic alteration in gene expression.

Diabetes

Diabetes can cause impotence due to impaired nerve function and blood vessels. In an article published in the *Journal of International Andrology*, Dr. Kapoor and colleagues in the UK reported that low testosterone levels and erectile dysfunction were frequently associated with type II diabetes. Even in diabetic men who had a normal level of total testosterone, the level of bio-available free testosterone (the form of testosterone that can be readily used by human body) could be low, which led to erectile dysfunction.

High level of blood cholesterol

When the level of low-density lipoprotein (bad cholesterol) is high and the level of high-density lipoprotein (good cholesterol) is low the endothelial (lining) and smooth muscle cells of the penis may be affected, leading to impaired erectile function. Oxidized low-density lipoprotein can also damage the relaxation response of the corpus cavernosum, a sponge-like tissue in penis. When the corpus cavernosum relaxes, it can hold sufficient blood to make solid erection.

Smoking and low-fat diet

Zmuda and colleagues in the University of Pittsburgh spent 13 years studying the relationship between total testosterone level, lifestyle, and behaviors. They observed 66 men aged 41-61 years-old. In their report published in 1977, they noticed that over the 13-year-study period people who smoked cigarettes showed more rapid decline in total testosterone than non-smokers. The more cigarettes people smoke, the more rapid the decline in their total testosterone level.

Heavy smoking also increases the level of sex binding protein, as suggested by Dr. English and colleagues of the

Royal Hallamshire Hospital of UK. Increased sex binding protein may decrease the level of bio-available testosterone. Another interesting finding in this study is that low-fat diet is also associated with a rapid decline of total testosterone in a group of people who tried to eat a low-fat diet over 10 to 13 years to prevent coronary heart disease. People who live a very healthy lifestyle with a vegan diet may have a healthier cardiovascular system, but if their testosterone level is too low, they will lose muscle mass and develop depression. I have been following up with many healthy 90- to 100-year-old seniors, of whom very few were on a vegan diet. Some vegan seniors look very healthy. I am not sure if their testosterone level is comparable to that of their non-vegan peers. I guess after 70 years of age, sex may not be so important for some men.

Behavior patterns

Generally speaking, behavior patterns can be divided into type A, type B and type AB. Type A personality exhibits intense, hard-driving competitiveness, a chronic sense of urgency, impatience, insecurity about one's status, aggressiveness, incapability of relaxation and easily evoked hostility. Type A behavior was first described as a potential risk factor in coronary disease in the 1950s by cardiologists Meyer Friedman and R. H. Rosenman. Type A individuals appear to respond to stress and challenges with an exaggerated increase in cortisol, which is known to suppress testosterone. The 13-year longitudinal study by Dr. Zmuda pointed out that type A behavior is associated with greater decline of total testosterone with aging. If a man wants to keep his optimal level of testosterone, he needs to relax periodically to bring the energy to his endocrine system.

Heart disease

When blood circulation is compromised, the functions of the testes will also be diminished. A study led by Dr. Kew-Kim Chew of Queen Elizabeth II Medical Center in Australia showed the increased risk of erectile dysfunction in men with cardiovascular diseases.

Erectile dysfunction has become a much-talked-about problem for middle-aged men with high stress jobs and a sedentary lifestyle. When men are in their twenties, their testosterone levels are naturally high, so they have stronger sexual drive and sexual function even under a lot of stress. If blood supply to the penis is sufficient and testosterone level is high, a man typically will not need strong stimulation in order to get an erection. After age 40, men's testosterone levels naturally go down a little bit every year. How fast erectile function declines depends on how healthy the man is, how well the man can manage his stress level, and how often he can have regular sex with his partner. I have treated erectile dysfunction in people who have had prostate surgery or have used blood pressure medication for long time. If a man can exercise every day, practice relaxation techniques such as yoga, meditation, Qi Gong, or reiki, and have acupuncture every two weeks, he can improve the energy flow to his lungs, heart, adrenal gland, thyroid gland, penis and testicles, which all help forestall the decline of testosterone. Research has verified that acupuncture can improve erectile dysfunction very effectively, especially for men with impotence due to stress and functional problems. Furthermore, acupuncture has none of the side effects of testosterone cream and injections, which can cause insomnia, excessive sweating, high blood pressure, anxiety, and enlarged prostate. For men who already have prostate inflammation or cancer, using artificial testosterone can be dangerous and may lead to relapse of the cancer.

Moreover, testosterone or even bio-identical hormones cannot improve the functions of the heart, lungs and testicles. On the other hand, testicular function can be weakened because the brain can detect the higher testosterone level and reduce the amount of luteinizing hormone (stimulating the testicular function) produced.

After a few years, a man's testicles may not function if he uses a high level of artificial testosterone. He may have more sexual drive or achieve orgasm more easily than before, but if he has to sacrifice his sleep, his patience, and the possibility of improving his testicular function more naturally, it is not worth trying.

I always tell my patients to try the natural way to improve their erectile function. First of all, you have to work with your partner. Having regular sex, not necessarily intercourse or achieving orgasm, two to three times a week can help both of you to reduce your stress level; it is free and the best sleeping pill you'll ever have. If you can make your partner sleep better at night, in the morning, you will see a smiling face, and sexual drive will increase over time. Life is short; we need to help our spouses be happy after a stressful day. If you try to have sex twice a week and are not satisfied with your performance, you can get acupuncture treatment once or twice a week for 10 treatments. You will find that your erectile function can quickly improve, and intercourse can become better and longer. When you resume regular sex, the brain cells become more sensitive to the stimulation and produce more stimulating hormones to make the pituitary and testicles create more sex-related hormones. More balanced hormones can help you cope with stress better and build stronger muscles. Your body and mind will form a positive cycle, and your whole life quality will be improved. Let us find healthy ways to become happier and healthier. Instead of taking pills, try a natural way to fix problems that has fewer side effects and costs a whole lot less.

Allergy treatment can lower blood testosterone level

A Bulgarian study of asthmatics treated with and without corticosteroids indicated that low blood testosterone was more frequent in the corticosteroid-treated patients than in patients who had never been treated with corticosteroids. Low blood testosterone was found mainly in the patients with a severe (37.76%) and moderate (40.00%) form of the disease and very rarely in patients with a mild form of bronchial asthma (8.51%). The testosterone level changes are probably due to stress, low oxygen, and corticosteroid treatment. The low oxygen level can lead to anxiety and panic attacks, which also contribute to impotence.

Poor nutrition and lack of regular sexual activities

In a report published in 2007 in the *Journal of Sex Medicine,* Dr. Ahn and colleagues in South Korea investigated the prevalence of erectile dysfunction and premature ejaculation in Korean men and the impact of general health, lifestyle, and psychosocial factors on these conditions. They interviewed 1,570 Korean men aged 40-79 years old with a self-administered questionnaire on sexual function and the International Index of Erectile Function. In addition, blood chemistry was analyzed for each subject. Their results indicated that erectile dysfunction was more prevalent in the subject groups with older age, lower income, or lower education, and in subjects without a spouse. Erectile dysfunction was positively associated with risk factors such as diabetes, hypertension, heart disease, psychological stress, and obesity. Levels of serum triglycerides, testosterone, or dehydroepiandrosterone sulfate (DHEA-S) were significantly different between the erectile dysfunction and normal groups.

Therefore, if men want to function the best when they get older, they need to have a happy relationship with their spouses or partners. Regular sex stimulates the brain to produce the optimal amount of stimulating hormone to the testes. The optimal amount of testosterone will help maintain testicular function. The U.S. Food and Drug Administration (FDA) estimates that 4 to 5 million American men may suffer from low testosterone, but only 5 percent of them are currently treated.

Symptoms of low testosterone

The common symptoms and signs of low testosterone include low sex drive and libido, erectile dysfunction, increased irritability or depression, fatigue, reduced muscle mass and strength, inability to concentrate, decreased bone density, sadness and grumpiness, quick deterioration in athletic and work performance, foggy headedness, or falling asleep after a big meal.

Researchers have shown that if a man is in perfect health, his testosterone can be within normal range at the age of eighty, even though it may be lower than when the man was in his twenties. He can still have normal sexual function, although it is not wise to have the same sexual behavior when a man reaches his seventies or eighties as he did in his twenties. For instance, if a man can have multiple sessions of intercourse in one day in his twenties or thirties, he should not do the same thing when he reaches eighty years old. Changing partners is not good for a man's health. Extremely fast, strong, and frequent sex can put a lot of burden on your heart and brain because when you have intercourse and orgasm, your heart rate and blood pressure increase dramatically and your blood is shunted to the penis. At the age of eighty, you should do everything slowly at a reasonable rate, so that your heart rate and blood pressure will not go so high as to cause a stroke or heart attack.

In the movie "Something's Got to Give", a sixty-year-old businessman with heart problems liked to have sex with young women in their twenties. He wanted to have as strong and fast an erection as a twenty-year-old man, so he took Viagra to bring more blood flow to his penis. The extreme excitement caused a sudden constriction of his heart blood vessels and sent him to the emergency room. What an embarrassment! Interestingly, his EKG was back to normal later. He had angina (chest pain) due to the over excitement with his young girlfriend. But if he keeps repeating this many times, eventually he will have permanent damage in his heart muscles because the heart muscle is very sensitive to the lack of oxygen. Of course, very exciting intercourse can bring many positive things: fleeting happiness, sometimes inspiration and creativity. Maybe this is one of the reasons that some writers and movie stars change their partners many times in their life. In this movie, when this businessman found a fifty-year-old, very successful woman with whom he could better communicate through common interests, his erection lasted longer without Viagra and the risk of heart attack. Furthermore, he was able to sleep through the night for the first time after many years of interrupted sleep. His relationship with this fifty-year-old woman ended, however, because he did not want to get married and he really loved those extremely exciting moments with younger women, even though he knew he might die of a heart attack.

Sometimes, trying to live the lifestyle of a younger person can speed up our demise. I once treated a 60-year-old man with high blood pressure and chronic insomnia. He had to get up in the middle of the night to take sleeping pill to help him fall back to sleep. He was diagnosed with bladder cancer and received chemotherapy. I checked his lifestyle and medical history and found he was divorced with one 25-year old son. He changed girlfriends frequently. He got so excited when he had sex with the new girlfriend that he had a hard time falling asleep or staying asleep. The rush of dopamine when you change partners every 6 months will stimulate your brain and change your sleep pattern. According to David Howard, when a person is in the early stages of a new relationship, his brain fires off dopamine, creating excitement. At the age of 60, the sleep pattern started changing. This man sacrificed his precious sleep time for the excitement of the new relationship, which can damage his health.

When we get older, our heart function, brain activity and blood circulation are all different than when we were in our twenties; we need to change our behavior accordingly. If you ask an eighty-year-old man to run a marathon, it is very likely to put him in a serious medical condition. But if you take good care of your health, you can still have normal sexual function at the age of ninety. Dr. Amen, a famous psychiatrist, told a story about a healthy ninety-year-old man who still planned to have sex with his wife after his hernia repairment surgery.

Furthermore, you have to be healthy in order to enjoy the moments the high testosterone brings to you, meaning your testosterone level has to match the function of other internal organs. Does high testosterone do all the good things to men's body? No, nothing is good if it is too much.

Age and testosterone

When men get older, certain enzymes and glandular function decline. If you are healthy, it is very likely your testosterone can stay within a normal functioning range, but lower than when you were 20 years old. Some researchers indicate that after the age of 40 to 50, men's testosterone level naturally decreases by 1% every year. At the age of 80, if a man is healthy, he can still have a normal range of testosterone and thus, the normal, age-matched sex life.

Using testosterone cream can influence your wife's health

Here is another story about how high testosterone can influence your family life. In the TV show, House, a middle-aged man had a very young girlfriend. He wanted to make his young girlfriend happy with their sex life. Instead of trying the hard way to be healthier to enhance his sexual behavior, he kept using artificial testosterone cream, thinking this magic cream could help him build strong muscles and optimize his sex life. The testosterone cream vaporized in the air and became absorbed by his daughter and his girlfriend. His daughter started her period at the age of 9 while his girlfriend started growing dark hair on her face. I think sex is very important, but a good relationship and mutual understanding can bring more happiness than strong sex.

Case study: vegan diet and low testosterone

Tom was born into a well-educated family in Boston. He went to a private high school in Westwood and graduated with very good grades. He followed his parents' advice and went to a premedical program at Brandeis University in

Waltham. Like other college students, he gained more than 20 lbs during the first two years. He also developed migraines and high cholesterol level due to inflammation of his blood vessels and nerves. Initially, he started taking anti-inflammatory medication such as ibuprofen. When the over-the-counter medication did not work anymore, he went to a migraine specialist at Newton-Wellesley Hospital and started the medication for migraine. The medication took away the pain but made him so tired and drowsy that he could not continue with his studies. Later, he had to take a year off and worked at a farm in Wellesley for a year because he could not study any more with debilitating headaches and depression. While he was working at the farm, he had the same food as the family did. For the whole year, he ate more vegetables and fruits and cut down on sweet and spicy foods, and of course, he did not have the chance to drink too much alcohol. Miraculously, his migraines got better and he was able to go back to study after a year. He was convinced that the vegetables and fruits provided sufficient minerals and vitamins to help him get rid of the inflammation. He gradually became vegan. At first, he still had some milk, cheese, or eggs, but later he got rid of all animal products.

After he graduated from college, he entered medical school at Tufts University in Boston. The four-year medical school training was very stressful; he lost 30 lbs with his vegan diet. Initially, he felt great. After one year in medical school, his energy level started going down, and he could barely stay awake after 10 pm. As a medical student, he had to work 60 hours a week. He did not have enough energy to work such a long time. Furthermore, he started losing his muscles even though he tried to lift weights. His digestion became a problem; he had bloating, gas, acid reflux and sometimes diarrhea. Finally, he decided to see an acupuncturist in Needham to figure out why his energy level was so low.

His acupuncturist recommended that he check his testosterone level and thyroid function at Boston Medical Center. It turned out that his testosterone level was below 300 and he developed a hypothyroid condition. After checking his medical history and diet, his acupuncturist recommended that he start eating one or two eggs each day. A vegan diet was good to clear up his inflammation, but a pure vegan diet required a perfect digestive system. The high stress level in medical school compromised his digestive function, and therefore, he could not absorb the proteins and vitamins from the vegan diet efficiently. He needed to eat some easily digestible proteins such as eggs or organic milk. Tom faithfully followed the instructions and had acupuncture treatments in the clinic twice a week for 2 months, followed by once a week for another month. His energy level came back and he was able to finish his four-year medical study and find a good residency program at Boston Medical Center.

Possible side effects of high testosterone level from the testosterone pill and cream

- Increased red blood cell number can cause thickening of the blood and blood clotting.

- Enlargement and cancer of the prostate.

- High blood pressure and sleep apnea.

- High cholesterol with acceleration of arteriosclerosis.

- Irritability and panic disorder.

- Aggressiveness.

- Excessive sweating with special odor.

- Insomnia.

Chapter 2

Natural Way to Optimize Your Testosterone Level

How to optimize a man's testosterone level

Avoid unnecessary medications. High blood pressure medication can not only influence erectile function, but also decrease sexual drive, according to James Goldberg, a pharmacologist in California. If you have high blood pressure, try to lose weight, cut down the salts, and eat less meat to lower the blood pressure first. With lifestyle changes, you can either avoid blood pressure medications or keep the dosage at the lowest functioning level. High blood pressure medications are designed to dilate the small blood vessels in your extremities; it becomes harder to achieve a normal erection if a lot of blood is accumulating in the peripheral areas and not circulating efficiently. You can reduce your stress and cut down your salt intake to lower your blood pressure in the early stages of the high blood pressure. You can also take some herbal tea, such as hibiscus tea, to lower your blood pressure.

Increase the amount of exercise in your daily routine. One study indicated that exercising three times a week enhances men's sexual drive by boosting the circulating testosterone level significantly compared to that of their couch potato counterparts. Also, the more lean muscle you have, the less your central fat and the higher your testosterone level. Body builders and men who do a lot of physical work hardly have impotence. It is the men who use their brain a lot that tend to develop impotence in their fifties or sixties. If men take too many medications or eat too much junk food, they can develop impotence even in their thirties. In the documentary *Supersize Me*, a man consistently ate supersized hamburgers and French fries and drank carbonated sodas for a month. He developed fatty liver and depression, gained 20 pounds, lost his sexual drive, and had temporary impotence in his twenties.

Regular sex life. If you are busy with work and kids, please try to find time to be with your partner. You will find out that after satisfying sex, your mental sharpness, work efficiency, and testosterone level can increase naturally. Most men can sleep deeper when they have regular sex with their wife or partner. Changing partners frequently is not good for the health. Interestingly, men and women have different physical responses after having sex: men feel exhausted and fall asleep faster while women feel stimulated and stay alert for a while.

Reduce your stress level. Try not to work or talk all the time. Take 20 to 30 minutes off to let your body and mind fully relax so that you can direct more blood flow to nourish your testis and adrenal gland. If you cannot stop thinking, you can try mindful meditation and acupuncture. Most people will fall asleep after insertion of the needles into their bodies during which the hormone levels will be optimized by balancing the reproductive energy. Tai Chi, Qi Gong and yoga can also help you reduce stress.

Avoid all simple sugars to optimize the insulin level. We know every time your blood sugar goes above a certain level, it will cause inflammation of the blood vessels, and damage your nerves, including the nerves that control sexual functions. That is why diabetes patients tend to have erectile dysfunction (ED) and prostate problems at an earlier age.

Studies have shown that some nutrients, especially vitamins A and E, zinc, and selenium can help correct androgen deficiency and enhance sperm production. Make sure you eat at least 5 servings of fruits and vegetables to get enough vitamins. Do not take too many vitamins or fish oil from food supplements. One study from the combined effort of University of Washington, the National Cancer Institute and Cleveland Clinic indicated that too much fish oil can increase the rate of prostate cancer. We should not worry about flax seed because there is so much fiber in them that you will not overeat this kind of whole foods. Omega-3 is good but do not take too much. I saw some body builders who took too much of different kinds of food supplements and ended up with prostate cancer. Some patients take too much fish oil every day and their PSA (prostate specific antigen) goes up abnormally. Whole foods are always better than food supplements.

Decrease alcohol consumption or quit alcohol completely. Consuming too much alcohol has been demonstrated to cause impotence and low testosterone level. Alcohol also damages your liver; then, your body will have more estrogen, which decreases your muscle mass and stimulates your breasts to grow. Also, too much estrogen can stimulate prostate growth. Alcohol can also make men convert testosterone into estrogen and speed up age-related decline of testosterone.

Furthermore, alcohol damages the nerves around the penis and causes neuropathy, the inflammation of the nerves.

After prostate surgery, the nerves around the penis can be damaged. You may want to start acupuncture treatment early to help restore the function of the peripheral nerves. The earlier you start treatment, the faster the nerves can regenerate. Electrical stimulation can speed up the regeneration of the nerves and bring the energy to your testes to produce more testosterone.

Try to have the right amount of good quality protein, such as fish, almonds and chicken. If your body does not have enough amino acid, it can also lead to low testosterone. Optimize your good fat intake. Long term low fat diet can accelerate the decline of testosterone in advanced age. Normal fat intake will not increase your total cholesterol. One of the most famous Chinese herbal practitioners had been a very strict vegan for over 30 years, ever since he was diagnosed with throat cancer. He religiously exercised every morning and never overate. His cancer was subsequently healed using a Chinese herbal formula. But in his writings, he made it clear that his family life was not perfect. I believe that he had lost his sex drive because of his diet over the years. In the end it affected his happiness significantly. He may lose muscles faster because of the low testosterone and may have depression.

If you wear jockey shorts, please switch to boxer-type underwear, which helps improve the blood flow to the testes. Riding a bike for hours is not good for your testicular function; Lance Armstrong had testicular cancer. Exercise is good, but too much of it can lead to a higher level of cortisol and lower testosterone level.

Avoid too much sex when you are young. In Chinese medicine, too much sex can damage your kidney function and make men develop impotence at earlier age. The last emperor of the Qing Dynasty of China started having sex with different concubines around 12 years old. By the age of thirty, he developed impotence. His servants tried so many methods to restore his sexual function, but the damage was too much. He never regained his normal function.

Acupuncture can help boost testosterone level by improving blood flow to the testes and by reducing stress hormones, such as cortisol. If you are a CEO with a very high level of stress, regular exercise and more sleep may not be sufficient to control your stress level. I recommend you have acupuncture at least once or twice a month even if you are currently in good health. After 40, your body will start changing. Pay more attention and spend more time taking care of your health so that when you reach 90, you will be able to enjoy life with optimal levels of different kinds of hormones.

Acupuncture and psychogenic erectile dysfunction

In one study, 22 men who had psychogenic erectile dysfunction were recruited. Twenty completed the study, including 10 patients after crossover (patients of the placebo group who subsequently received acupuncture treatment). A satisfactory response was achieved in 68.4% of the acupuncture treatment group and in 9% of the placebo group. Another 21.05% of the patients of the treatment group had improved erections of similar rigidity to those taking Viagra. Acupuncture was an effective treatment option in more than two-thirds of these patients with psychogenic erectile dysfunction.

A Korean scientist, H.G. Kho did a pilot study of 16 patients suffering from ED. Using acupuncture only to treat erectile dysfunction did not influence the profile of stress and sex hormones, but did improve the quality of erections and restored sexual activity with an overall 39% effective rate. In another study, F. Fischl used acupuncture to treat 28 men with sub-clinical infertility. Each patient received a total of 10 treatments for a period of three weeks. In all cases, there was a statistically significant improvement of sperm total count, concentration, and motility.

For diabetes patients, if you are in your forties or fifties, acupuncture has been verified to help regenerate the peripheral nerves including the nerve controlling the testes and bladder. The treatment may take a few months and should be combined with weight control, diet, and lifestyle changes. If your blood sugar continues to be high after each unhealthy meal, having acupuncture every day can only slow down your nerve degeneration to a certain point because every time your blood sugar goes up, your nerves and blood vessels get damaged. So, whenever you eat chocolate or put sugar in your coffee, please say to yourself: "I am putting this toxin into my body to ruin my sexual life just for a short period of enjoyment."

In a study carried out in the Chengdu University of Traditional Chinese Medicine in China, researchers used one kind of chemical-induced diabetes rat model. The rats were divided into 3 groups: a group of diabetic ED received no treatment, a group of diabetic ED received moxibustion (burning the herb called mugwort above certain points), and a control group of normal rats. The moxibustion group was treated at "Shenshu" (BL 23, 1.5 cun lateral to the lower border of the spinous process of the 2nd lumbar vertebra) and "Sanyinjiao" (SP6, 3 cun superior to medial malleolus) with small moxa cone about the size of a wheat grain. The results showed that moxibustion helped lower blood sugar, and more significantly, increased the amount of a chemical called nitric oxide in the penis to enhance erectile function.

Why do some practitioners get better results than others?
The following study carried out by M. Inoue et al. of Japan may help answer this question. They examined the effects of electro-acupuncture with direct current (DC) on peripheral nerve regeneration. The left sciatic nerve of 55 seven-month-old rats was crushed at the thigh. The rats were randomly allocated to four groups: distal cathode direct current group (n = 15), distal anode direct current group (n = 14), sham-operated group (n = 13), and control group (n = 13). In the distal cathode direct current group, a cathode electrode (positive) was connected to an insulated acupuncture needle inserted at 1 cm distal to the injured site, while an anode

electrode (negative) was connected to a needle inserted at 1 cm proximal to the lesion. In the distal anode direct current group, the order was reversed. In the sham-operated group, no electrical stimulation was given to the insulated needle inserted at the same sites. In the control group, no treatment was given.

Regeneration of peripheral nerves was faster in the distal cathode DC group than in the other groups, while in the distal anode DC group, the regeneration was delayed. This result suggested that electro-acupuncture with cathode (positive) electrode distal to the injury site might be a useful treatment with the advantage of enabling damaged tissue to repair faster because the negative electrode tends to have stronger electrical current. Clinically, the positive electrode delivers different stimulation compared to anode (negative) electrode. One theory indicates that the cathode electrode has a relaxing effect, whereas the anode electrode has a stimulating effect. Clinically, when two needles are connected to two electrodes, most of the time, the patient only feels a vibration on the negative electrode side. Considering that the part closest to the damaged tissue needs to be stimulated whereas the distal (further away) part needs a more relaxing effect so that more blood can flow to the distal injury, this research result makes sense for nerve regeneration.

Another relevant study was published in 2007 in the *European Journal of Neurology* by Schröder and colleagues of the Heidelberg School of Chinese Medicine in Germany. In this study, 192 patients with peripheral neuropathy as diagnosed by nerve conduction studies (NCS) were evaluated over a period of one year. Of the 47 patients who met the criteria for peripheral neuropathy of undefined etiology, 21 patients received acupuncture therapy according to classical Chinese medicine as defined by the Heidelberg Model, while the other 26 patients received the best medical care available but no specific treatment for peripheral neuropathy. Sixteen patients (76%) in the acupuncture group improved symptomatically and objectively, as measured by nerve conduction studies, while only four patients in the control group (15%) did so. Importantly, subjective improvement was fully correlated with improvement in nerve conduction studies in both groups. These data provided objective measurements to prove that acupuncture does help improve the peripheral nerve function. This study also indicated that acupuncture can help lower blood sugar and blood lipids, increase nerve conduction, and reduce blood viscosity and internal bleeding.

ED and macular degeneration

Macular degeneration is an age-related vision problem. The part of the retina which is responsible for central vision has many nerve cells and blood vessels. If you want to keep your vision in relatively good condition when you reach 90 years old, you need to have healthy blood vessels and nerves. If you consume too much salt and sugar every day and do not have sufficient exercise, your blood vessels and optic nerves will not function well. The aging of your retina will accelerate. The other organ which similarly has a lot of nerves and blood vessels is the penis. Only if a man has very healthy blood vessels and nerve cells can he have a strong erection. That is why impotence and macular degeneration share many similarities.

R. Klein et al. published a paper in the *American Journal of Ophthalmology* in 2004 indicating that macular degeneration and impotence have similar risk factors, such as diabetes, hypertension, stroke, chronic kidney disease, sleep apnea, alcohol intake, smoking, low testosterone, hyperparathyroidism, atherosclerosis, high cholesterol and cardiovascular disease. All of those risk factors can compromise the blood flow to your retina, testicles, joints, and brain. In order to avoid those conditions, you need eat more fruits and vegetables and avoid the factors causing inflammation of the blood vessels and nerves, such as spicy food, high salt, high sugar, and too much alcohol, dark chocolate, or nuts.

Dr. Harun Cakmak and colleagues conducted research on the relationship between neovascular age-related macular degeneration and ED. They found that 64.8% of the control group had some degree of ED and, of them, 31.4% had severe ED. In the group with neovascular macular degeneration, 94.6% had some degree of ED and, of them, 55.6% had severe ED

Why do people who suffer ED have a higher chance of developing macular degeneration? Costa and Virag explained the mechanism in a paper titled "The endothelial-erectile dysfunction connection" published in 2009 in the *Journal of Sexual Medicine*. According to Costa and Virag, insufficient nitric oxide (NO) can contribute to endothelial dysfunction. If NO is insufficient, the blood vessels cannot dilate sufficiently, and people tend to develop high blood pressure, Reynaud's, arthritis, migraine, and impotence. If people stay inside for too long with no time to relax and take a deep breath, their NO will be insufficient, and their blood vessels will constrict chronically. That is why people who are physically active and work outdoors have less ED and macular degeneration. The energy flow to their retina and penis is much better than in people who sit in front of a computer for more than 6 hours a day. Intense exercises will help push the blood to your brain, eyes, and extremities. People always tell me that after intense exercise, their vision seems better.

Acupuncture, meditation, or just simply breathing deeply will increase your NO instantly. In order to avoid ED and macular degeneration in your early forties, you need to do more physical exercise and get acupuncture treatment once a week even if you have no ED currently. At the end of the day, before you go to sleep, you can meditate for 15 min to increase your NO concentration and dilate your blood vessels, including the blood vessels in the eyes, joints, and testicles.

Chapter 3

How Acupuncture can Help ED

Case 1: Low testosterone, enlarged prostate, and normal sexual function

Gary was brought to Boston by his parents when he was a teenager. He was very smart but did not like to study. He worked with his father to maintain a small business in the Dedham area. Heavy lifting along with a diet high in sugar and salt contributed to his developing varicose veins around his testicles and lower abdominal area. Because he had very strong muscles due to his physical work, his testosterone had been very high. He worked hard and played hard as a truck driver in the Greater Boston area. When he was in his early twenties, he would have intercourse 2 to 3 times a day with his girlfriend. By age 30, his sexual drive was still good, but his sperm count was very low. His extended family was used to having a large number of children, and he desperately wanted to have more than one child. By the time he got married and bought a house, his doctor told him that he could not have children the natural way.

His urologist in Newton told him that he needed surgery to get rid of his varicose veins so that his sperm could survive longer with the lower temperature around his testicles. He took a chance and had two surgeries to correct the varicose veins around his testicular and lower abdominal area. The surgeries did not help his infertility but damaged so many nerves that he developed urinary retention. At the age of 50, his sexual drive declined so much that he could have sex only once a month and his testosterone level was around 370 ng/dL. He also had to get up 3 to 4 times a night to urinate. His prostate was enlarged and his PSA kept going up from 1 to 8 ng/mL.

He had tried many food supplements for three years, but his PSA could not be lowered. Finally, he decided to try acupuncture and Chinese herbs. He started acupuncture treatment at Boston Chinese Acupuncture twice a week for a few months. He first noticed that his urine flow became stronger after 3 months of treatment. Then, he started Chinese herbs. After 6 months of acupuncture and Chinese herbs, his testosterone level went up to 750 ng/dL, which is in the normal range for his age. Also, his PSA dropped to 4 ng/mL. He did not need to get a biopsy from his urologist in Boston. His impotence went away, and he could have sex twice a week. His erection could last more than 20 minutes with Chinese herbs and acupuncture once a week. The herbs helped lower his stress level and his testicles produced more testosterone. His sleep became deeper, and he only needed to get up 1 to 2 times per night. His energy level also increased a lot.

Case 2: Low testosterone, weight loss, joint pain, and perfect sexual function after acupuncture treatment

Mr. Levy was born in Boston and started college at Boston University when he was 18 years old. He was a wild young man. He got a young lady pregnant after meeting her at a bar the first time he was allowed to drink. He was raised in a very responsible family and was determined to be responsible for his son. He sent money to his girlfriend for child support when he served in the army in Florida. He had had a very strong sexual drive before he reached 45 years of age. He bragged that he could have intercourse 4 times per day between the ages of 18 and 35. Of course, he loved to drink alcohol and eat sweets.

By the time he reached his forties, his testosterone had dropped to 300 ng/dL, and his sexual drive plunged. He had severe knee pain and jaw pain due to inflammation. He changed his behavior as he became older. In his forties, he found a very attractive and responsible girlfriend. He was surprised that his erection was insufficient, even though he found a beautiful woman whom he really loved. That was one of the reasons he came to Boston Chinese Acupuncture in Needham to seek acupuncture treatment.

The acupuncturist first went through his diet and lifestyle to figure out why he had low testosterone and impotence. He had gained more than 30 pounds during the last 20 years. With the fat accumulating around his belly, his testosterone gradually dropped because estrogen is mainly stored in fat, which is why a man with a big belly tends to develop impotence. He also drank beer and wine daily at home. The alcohol further drove his estrogen level up and testosterone level down because his liver could not deactivate the estrogen. Furthermore, his high-stress job made his testosterone decline even more. His acupuncturist recommended exercise to build stronger muscles and higher levels of testosterone. He cut down on alcohol and sweets. In the meantime, he started drinking green juice and getting acupuncture treatments for impotence. After 24 electro-acupuncture treatments once or twice a week, this former army man lost 15 lbs, his knee pain went away, and he could then have intercourse more than 3 times a week. His increased endurance made him and his future wife very happy.

Case 3: Young man does not need penis transplant

Many factors can contribute to impotence. Aging is one of the main factors. If a man is healthy, his testosterone will drop 1% each year after he passes 50 or 60 years of age. Men with diabetes lose their sexual function much faster than other men, because their testicular function is compromised by the inflammation of their blood vessels and nerves. Most men with diabetes, high blood pressure or high blood cholesterol develop ED much earlier than healthy men.

Blood vessels and nerves are your network systems; every organ needs sufficient blood flow and nerve control to function normally. If a man has been eating processed foods loaded with salt and fructose since childhood, by the age of 30, the majority of his network is damaged. Of course, the body can regenerate nerves and blood vessels, but the speed of regeneration starts to slow down after 25 years of age, especially if a man does not exercise or eat enough vegetables. Here is an example of how a 27-year-old man almost got a penis transplant.

Karl is a programmer from India. Like many other computer geniuses in his company in Delray Beach, he loved to drink soda. He moved to Pompano Beach from Fort Lauderdale two years ago because of the better morning commute. It is difficult to drive to Delray Beach in the morning, and he tended to go to bed late and get up late. After sitting in front of a computer for more than 8 hours a day, at his Pompano Beach home, he ate sweets and enjoyed computer games. Five years after he moved to America, he gained 20 pounds, and his handsome face acquired a double chin. Then, he discovered that he had developed impotence at the age of 26. Initially, he still had a morning erection when his bladder was full. One year later, the morning erection was gone. He went to an urologist at Boynton Beach Hospital to get his penis and testosterone checked. His urologist recommended that he get a penis transplant at the age of 27.

He was very upset and came to Boca Raton Acupuncture Clinic to see if he could get a holistic treatment. His acupuncturist collected all his medical information and examined his pulse and tongue. He was told he had Qi and blood stasis, meaning his energy flow was blocked due to lack of exercise. His sublingual veins were purple and enlarged, indicating that his blood vessels and nerves were not functioning well. That is why he stopped having morning erections at the young age. He also recalled that he injured himself as a teenager while riding a bike. His acupuncturist told him that it would take a few months to recover the normal function of his blood vessels and nerves. In the meantime, he needed to eat a lot of fruits and vegetables because vitamins and minerals are critical for rebuilding a healthy network. He had a fiancée in India and planned to get married soon, so he was very motivated to fix his impotence. He came for acupuncture twice a week for 3 months, then once a week for 6 more months. Gradually, his morning erection came back. After a year of acupuncture treatments, he went back to Boynton Beach Hospital and got his testosterone level tested. The testosterone had gone up from 300 ng/dL to 800 ng/dL, and he recovered his normal erectile function. He got married a few months later.

Case 4: High blood pressure, high cholesterol and ED

David had high blood pressure and high blood cholesterol for many years. He had been taking Lipitor and blood pressure medications for more than five years. When he first started taking blood pressure medications, he developed impotence. His beautiful wife thought he might not be interested in her anymore. He mentioned this to his physician and tried different kinds of blood pressure medications. Finally, he found the right blood pressure pill, which allowed him to keep his sexual function. Occasionally, if his stress level became too high, he would develop temporary impotence. His main complaint was muscle pain in his upper and lower back and prostate problems. His muscle pain was always located at the same spot, indicating some kind of chronic inflammation instead of just a muscle sprain. Interestingly, swimming did not help the pain at all, even though he felt very relaxed afterwards.

He felt better after each acupuncture treatment for the muscle pain, but the pain would come back shortly afterwards. It seems that there was an underlying problem causing those muscle aches. This was the first time I started suspecting the drug Lipitor. David really enjoyed sweets and was not willing to change his diet, so he would rather continue taking Lipitor to lower his cholesterol. He was diagnosed with prostatic hyperplasia at the age of 55, when he suddenly could not urinate after he came back from a vacation. He was sent to the emergency room and had a catheter put into his bladder. The urologist said his prostate enlargement was moderate, which should not cause urination problems for other people.

When he was very young, he worked in a very remote area without a restroom close by, so he used to hold his urine for many hours during the day. Of course, he would also not drink water. This may have caused his bladder muscle to lose its elasticity after many years of over-stretching.

Furthermore, the lack of water intake could lead to urinary tract infection. Before he had acute urine retention, his bladder muscle had already become weaker. One time, while traveling, after sitting in an airplane for a long time and taking cold medication, his bladder muscle suddenly stopped functioning. This acute urine retention problem had happened many times. David finally decided to do something to fix the problem.

We started acupuncture treatment on his lower abdominal and back areas. When he had constipation, his urine retention got worse with increased frequency and urgency. One time when he went to Mexico for a vacation, I gave him a Chinese herbal formula, and his urination and constipation dramatically improved. Due to his continued use of blood pressure medications that influence his bladder muscle, however, the problem periodically returned. Finally, he was convinced that partially abrading his prostate by laser surgery was the only way to solve his problem. We assumed that if his problems were due to an enlarged prostate, the frequent urination and urine retention should be fixed after surgery. As a routine, he had a catheter put in during and after surgery. Because his bladder muscle became weaker with the catheter, he could not urinate for a while, and his urine frequency increased after surgery. I told him that we needed to strengthen his bladder muscle, so that he could empty his bladder more efficiently and prevent infection.

We did 10 treatments after his catheter was removed. He was able to urinate normally by himself after only one treatment. With acupuncture treatment once or twice a month for a couple of years after the surgery, his constant urgency to urinate became less intense. With strengthened bladder muscles, the residual urine in his bladder dramatically decreased. His urgency to urinate also was reduced due to the lessened inflammation of his bladder and urethra. He continued with all of his medications and acupuncture treatments for many years, but his tongue very often showed a thick greasy coating, indicating digestive inefficiency, which can cause urination problems. We used herbs to improve his digestion. After surgery, his physician put him on Diazepam to make him less anxious. His impotence got worse, so we focused on improving his testosterone level and erectile function. Finally, he stopped Diazepam and Flomax, a commonly used medication to relax the bladder muscle. With the acupuncture treatments, his impotence was gone. Ten months after his prostate surgery, he had another urine retention attack in June 2002. We had to do another 10 acupuncture treatments to bring back his normal urination. Acupuncture helped restore his normal urination function each time his problem was triggered by stress, cold, or other problems. In June 2005, he developed kidney stones. The pain was so severe that he vomited bile and almost fainted. He drank tea every day because he thought, the more antioxidants he took, the better.

I have been treating this gentleman for more than 16 years. I did not see any dramatic change after the laser surgery on his prostate. He still has acute urination retention once or twice a year. Sometimes, he has blood in his urine, which scared him to death at first. In my opinion, if he had stopped eating simple sugars, lowered his cholesterol by changing his lifestyle, and cut down his medications, he might have been able to improve his bladder function more. Stress was another trigger aggravating his urine problem. One time when he needed to fast for 24 hours for a blood test, his urine retention came back instantly. So far, his urine retention problem has not been completely solved, but his ED problem is getting better with regular acupuncture treatment.

Case 5: Injection of testosterone can lead to high blood pressure and high eye pressure

Mr. George Yang was born into a well-educated family near Boston. With hard work and connections, he got into Harvard University and graduated 40 years ago. He has become a prolific and famous writer over the past twenty years. With the advent of computers, his writing speed has become faster and faster. He published many important articles in influential newspapers in the Boston area. However, his eyesight started changing when he turned 50, and his prostate became inflamed with daily consumption of alcohol. Many writers think they can get inspiration while drinking alcohol. That may be true, but the alcohol not only damaged his neurons and prostate, but also damaged another important network: his blood vessels. Once the blood vessels and nerves were inflamed, prostate cancer, eye problems, and impotence arrived one after another.

Mr. Yang came to Boston Chinese Acupuncture initially to seek help for his increased eye pressure, which was around 20 to 23 mmHg. As a famous writer, losing his vision could be devastating to his career. The acupuncturist started using a specific protocol to relax his neck and eye muscles. After 3 months, Mr. Yang went back to a hospital and got his pressure checked again. Surprisingly, his eye pressure dropped to 17. His dry eye problem got better, and his vision improved.

After his eye pressure went down, he started having acupuncture once a week instead of twice a week. While his acupuncturist continued to treat his eye problem, he mentioned that he would like to improve his sexual function. He had had his prostate removed a few years back due to prostate cancer. After the surgery, he developed impotence. Initially, he was getting testosterone injections, but later, he found out that the testosterone injections made his blood pressure go up, which also might have increased his eye pressure. He finally decided to stop the testosterone injections and started getting acupuncture to improve his ED. He also cut down his alcohol to once a week instead of every day, which helped him sleep deeply. After a year of acupuncture treatments, his ED improved.

In 2016, Mr. Yang had cataract surgery; and his eye pressure went up again to 23 mmHg. He decided to buy a very expensive machine to monitor his eye pressure daily. His acupuncturist recommended that he have acupuncture twice a week for a few weeks until his eye pressure stabilized. His acupuncturist also recommended that he do acupressure every morning and night, and then measure his eye pressure with his fancy machine in the morning. His eye pressure usually went up in the morning even though he had used eye drops and practiced acupressure the night before. He then tried meditating at the same time as when he was doing his acupressure in the morning. After half an hour, he measured his eye pressure again; it dropped from 22 to 18 mmHg. If he had an acupuncture treatment, his eye pressure sometimes would drop even lower for a few days. He now practices acupressure together with meditation and has acupuncture treatment every two weeks to maintain his vision and testosterone level.

Case 6: ED, hair loss and drooping eye lids

Mr. Rosenthal came to Boston Chinese Acupuncture for a stomach problem. At the initial appointment, I learned that in addition to stomach cramps and knee pain, he suffered from panic attacks periodically. He told me that he had a high stress managerial position in a high-tech company and that he felt a bit out of control on occasion. I understood generally what he was telling me; however, I could tell at that point that he had other health problems that he didn't feel comfortable sharing. By his manner and my observations, I was convinced that he had not told me the whole story.

As I treated him, I found out more. He had been a serious runner all his life and had arthritis in his knee for 10 years. Stomach issues plagued him since childhood. Whenever he skipped a meal or got nervous about something, he would have severe stomach pain. He mentioned that recently, he developed rashes on his torso. At the fifth visit, I found out what he had been unwilling to talk about. He was too reserved a man and so much a product of his socially conservative New England upbringing.

Mr. Rosenthal told me that he had never shared this with anyone else, not even his wife. Early in his fifties, he noticed that his high sex drive was gone. It depressed him and caused him to lose energy in a general way. He went to see his urologist and found out that his testosterone level was down at the lower end of the normal range. He started testosterone cream externally, hoping to save his libido and improve the quality of his sex life. With his stressful job, he could not sleep well, waking up around 4 AM, and developed night sweats and dizziness. His feet have poor circulation generally, and he loves having one or two glasses of wine during dinner time. He mentioned that his sleep could be interrupted by his alcohol intake. When I first met Mr. Rosenthal, he mentioned that he always felt hot at room temperature and was constantly sweating.

I started clearing the blocked heat in his upper and lower body using acupuncture. After only three treatments, his stomach problems affected him less frequently, while he continued taking herbal powder from a naturopathic doctor. His panic attacks lessened, and his knee pain abated. After three more treatments, he could have lunch with business partners without worrying about stomach cramps. His sleep, although not perfect, was improving. I was very surprised by his quick response and thought that maybe he was on a tight budget, so we cut down his treatments to once a month. It seemed that the once-a-month treatment was able to help his body optimize its digestive function. After five treatments, he got his testosterone retested: it had almost doubled. In the meantime, he had more spontaneous sweating with increased blood pressure. I suggested that he cut down his testosterone gel to every other day. During the summer, his blood pressure decreased with reduced use of testosterone cream, and his face was not as red as before.

In November 2007, I treated him twice with neck and back points while he was lying face-down to relieve the tightness in those areas. He could then sleep for 6 straight hours. He maintained monthly treatments, and gradually, his sleep became deeper and sometimes lasted for seven hours.

When the economy started to dive in 2008, his testosterone dropped dramatically because his stress level increased, even with very good sleep. He increased the testosterone dosage to save his libido again. I suggested that he switch to bioidentical testosterone if he had to use hormones. His sleep would increase to seven hours right after acupuncture treatment but gradually went back to five hours within two weeks. He then increased the frequency of treatments to every two weeks. Surprisingly, his old allergies came back, and he could not lay face-down to have treatment on his stomach. He mysteriously stopped treatments for a month; I figured he might have some other issues.

When he finally called a month after his last treatment in October, he reported that he had developed eye tearing right after the last acupuncture treatment. His left eye turned red, with tears coming down his face, especially in the morning. His left eye was also constantly producing pus. Afterwards, his eye would become very dry. I suggested that he see an ophthalmologist. In the meantime, he perspired a lot during the treatment. I attributed his eye problems to his alcohol intake and possible blockage of his tear ducts. Consumption of alcohol produced a lot of internal heat, especially in his liver channel, which was associated with the redness and tearing of his left eye. The checkup showed inflammation of the left eye and drooping of the lower eyelid. His ophthalmologist suggested surgery to remove part of his eyelid.

I suggested he postpone the surgery and try acupuncture and herbs first for a couple of months to see if we could relieve the symptoms. He started once-a-week treatments in December. In the meantime, I was trying to convince him to cut down his red wine intake. His red eye went away after 4 treatments. At this point, he finally decided to stop the testosterone cream because his blood pressure was constantly high. With once-a-week acupuncture treatments, his sexual drive started to improve at the age of 55.

He still drank one glass of red wine every night with his meal. I noticed that his feet had poor circulation with constant sweating, coldness, and hyper-sensitivity when I used alcohol to clean his feet. He argued that this was genetic because his dad also had the same hyper-reflex. His tongue had many purple spots, and the sublingual vein looked enlarged and purple. Two months after acupuncture treatments for his eyes, his tearing was reduced and did not run down his face, but he still had to use antibiotic eye drops. Finally, he stopped drinking wine during the week because he was worried that his testosterone would go down again after he stopped using testosterone cream. We started Chinese herbal treatment. After three weeks, his eye pus decreased, so that he only needed to use antibiotic eye drops every three to four days. Furthermore, his sleep became much deeper after he stopped drinking alcohol during the week. He also cut down on sweets and coffee, which made him much calmer to cope with difficult situations without panic attacks.

With only acupuncture once a week, I was able to reduce the tears in his left eye so that it did not run down his face very often. His sleep became very deep, but the pus came and went. I then recommended that he take Chinese herbs. After taking herbs for four months, his tear production became normal with no pus coming out. He only occasionally needed to use eye drops. The purple spots on his tongue disappeared and the redness of his face was reduced. Furthermore, the hyper-reflex on his left foot went away, indicating a more balanced nervous system. He did not have a panic attack since he started acupuncture treatment.

In this case, Mr. Rosenthal's daily stress, indigestion, and intake of alcohol, sweets, and coffee, together with aging, led to his low testosterone, so that he started losing libido and muscle mass. The artificial testosterone he was given caused him to have accelerated hair loss. To save his hair, he was given Propecia, which caused his eyelid muscle to droop. Why did it happen to his left eye but not his right? Maybe it was the old injury occurred when he boxed in his twenties. He scheduled an eye operation in June 2008. The combination of Chinese herbs and weekly acupuncture treatments, however, enabled him to cancel the surgery and save the risk of the procedure and the time he would have lost.

The two cups of coffee he drank in the morning increased his heart rate and blood pressure dramatically. He later cut down the coffee to one cup. He gradually cut down his alcohol intake to once a week. After reducing his alcohol intake, he felt more refreshed in the morning and the purple spot on his tongue gradually disappeared. He was able to stop the antibiotic eye drops after taking herbs for six months. Interestingly, he observed that taking apple cider vinegar helped reduce the pus in his eyes, but his sleep decreased to 6 hours. When his stress level increased, his eye produced more pus.

Case 7: Low testosterone, hypothyroidism, and impotence

Steven was a software programmer. He came to the acupuncture clinic mainly for right shoulder pain when he was 27-year old. From a medical point of view, at this age, his hormones should be at a peak level. He should not have any age-related degenerative diseases. His job required him to sit in front of a computer for a long time. Like many single guys, he ate a lot of processed foods, soda, and sweets. One day he suddenly could not get up from bed. His energy was so low that he could not think correctly. He made a lot of money by doing computer work, but not enough to stop working at this point. He went to see his primary care physician (PCP) and hoped the doctor could help him figure out what was wrong with him.

Blood biochemistry showed that his thyroid hormones were very low, his testosterone was around 300 ng/dL, and his total cholesterol was over 300 mg/dL. He also had the additional nasty problems for a man of his age: decreased urine flow and, tragically, impotence. His PCP started him on Synthroid to boost his thyroid function. He did have enough energy to work, but his erections did not show any improvement. He also had new symptoms: frequent night urination, palpitations, and sweating when he was stressed. He became very anxious about trivial things, such as whether he could find the restroom right away.

He also noticed that when he was with his girlfriend, he could not get an erection. He went to an urologist to get his ED fixed. He went through all the urological tests. One of the tests involves injecting saline into his penis to see if the blood will flow normally. Originally, he had typical morning erections when his bladder was full. After he went through the exhaustive testing, his morning erection disappeared for some reason. His urologist recommended surgery in which part of the tissue in his penis would be removed and some artificial material implanted in his penis. He had already gone through all these tests with much discomfort, so finally, he decided to try something else. He asked me if he should do the surgery. I recommend that he try other methods first.

Since he had lost his morning erection for the past couple of months, I thought there might be some nerve injury involved. He later told me that he did injure his penis area when he tried to jump down from a high place at the age of 10. I recommended that he not ride his bike for a while and wear looser underwear. Then, we started using acupuncture to treat his shoulder pain along with his impotence problem. In order to help peripheral nerve regeneration, I did a localized acupuncture treatment, combining it with hormone balancing. After 12 treatments, he gradually got his morning erection back, but when his stress level increased or he did not sleep well, the morning erection started to wane. Since he did not have a steady girlfriend at that time, he could not test to see if he could have intercourse. We changed the acupuncture treatment to twice a month to continue improving the blood circulation and nerve function after his initial 12 treatments. Gradually, his impotence showed signs of improvement. After a year, he met a girl and they became friends. After a time, they got engaged. His treatments continued, and his impotence completely disappeared. When I spoke to him later, he told me that it had been the right decision not to have the surgery.

Case 8: Pituitary Gland and Low Testosterone

Mr. Lee was born in Boston and graduated from a college in Boston with an engineering degree. Since childhood, Mr. Lee had been a very energetic person, always having an optimistic, positive approach towards life and work. After graduation, he soon found a job in downtown Boston, and became accustomed to simultaneously managing many projects; the more challenging the projects, the more energized and stimulated he felt. He found it difficult performing boring tasks, and had been diagnosed with ADHD in his early twenties. He refused to take ADHD medication; instead, he would run 6 miles every other day and swim for an hour the rest of week. Intense exercise always helped him focus more on the boring tasks. He was promoted within his company, and married a lovely young woman in Wellesley, Massachusetts. Soon they moved to California because his wife found a better job in California.

A few years after Mr. Lee left Boston, he suddenly developed difficulty breathing; his lungs were irritated, and his brain was not as sharp as before. He also developed erectile dysfunction. His testosterone level dropped below 200 ng/dL. He also quickly lost muscle mass. He could no longer work as a head of an engineering team in California.

He needed support from his parents in Boston, and clear diagnoses from specialists. He visited many physicians in Boston and was diagnosed with pituitary gland insufficiency, because he had been exposed to mold in his house for too long, while living in California. The allergic reaction to mold led to water accumulation in his lungs, and toxic encephalopathy. The inflammation of his brain compromised his pituitary gland function, reducing the production of stimulating hormones to the testicles and adrenal gland. With very low testosterone level, Mr. Lee developed brain fog, fatigue, and ED.

In order to keep his muscle tone and erectile function, his physician started giving him weekly testosterone injections, hoping that would help him gain back his muscle tone, and resolve his ED problem. After receiving testosterone injections once a week for a few weeks, his blood viscosity increased significantly. Because he had experienced high blood pressure for many years, his doctor was concerned that he might suffer a stroke; hence the frequency of the testosterone injections was reduced to once every 4 weeks. The artificial testosterone made his ADHD worse; he had a hard time focusing on even a single project, and his brain would jump from one subject to another. Eventually, he cut down the testosterone injections to every 12 weeks.

He also tried Viagra, which made his erection abnormally strong, and damaged his penis. His penis developed a curvature when he had erection.

Finally, his lovely wife recommended that he take an herb called citrulline to help his ED. Combining citrulline and testosterone injections, he was able to have normal intercourse once or twice a week. However, after 12 weeks, he felt very tired, and had a hard time maintaining his normal work flow.

When he came to the clinic of Boston Chinese Acupuncture, he was planning to continue testosterone injections every two weeks. His energy level was low, and he had gained weight. His erection was not as strong as before. As the last resort, Mr. Lee wanted to try acupuncture to improve his testicular, and pituitary gland function.

The acupuncturist applied electrical acupuncture stimulation on certain areas of his scalp, and abdominal areas, hoping that acupuncture could bring more blood flow to his pituitary gland, and testes, so that he could produce more natural testosterone himself. After 4 acupuncture treatments, Mr. Lee gained so much energy that he was able to resume managing multiple projects at the same time as he did before he became sick. In the meantime, he achieved a stronger and longer erection even after he had stopped taking citrulline for a few days. The curvature of his penis was reduced, compared to that before acupuncture treatment. His increased energy level also allowed him to increase his exercise routine, resulting in weight loss.

If he continues acupuncture treatment for a few months, he may be able to enhance the functions of pituitary gland and testes. He may also be able to cut down his testosterone injection to every 16 or 20 weeks, which can reduce his risk of developing stroke and prostate cancer.

Chapter 4

Chinese Herbs, Testosterone, and ED

Testosterone has a wide normal range: from 300 to 900 ng/dL. An 80-year-old man can have testosterone around 500 ng/dL, while a 20-year-old can have 350 ng/dL. Impotence is not just associated with testosterone level. The functions of nerves and blood vessels can also play important roles. Physically active men tend to have strong erections and healthier blood vessels and nerves if they have a healthy diet. I treated a man who had gone through many surgeries for varicose veins and also had a lower testosterone level, but he ate very healthy foods and could still have normal erections. On the other hand, some men who consume just one glass of alcohol and one small piece of cookie every day have compromised nerve and blood vessel function. They tend to develop aneurisms, neuropathy, and high cholesterol. If they take blood pressure medication at the same time, they tend to have ED and urine retention, especially after prostate surgery.

With Chinese herbs, we can lower blood sugar level, reduce visceral fat, and help the body produce more growth hormones and testosterone. Kidney-tonifying herbs are especially helpful in building stronger muscles and maintaining higher levels of testosterone. Yin Yang Huo (Herba epimedium or horny goat weed) is one of the herbs that can help men improve their sexual function. I use Yin Yang Huo to help women and men balance their hormones. Yin Yang Huo has other good effects for improving joint function, opening the channels, and expelling wind cold for arthritis and joint pain.

A company made Yin Yang Huo tablets for men, but this is not a healthy way to treat ED. Yin Yang Huo is warm in quality. It can make the body produce too much heat if not used with other balancing herbs. In Chinese medicine, we put different herbs together to reduce their side effects and enhance their therapeutic effects. If a man takes too much Yin Yang Huo, he can potentially damage his kidney Yin, which can cause inflammation in the prostate, urinary tract infection, and even premature ejaculation. In the cases of impotence which I have treated in the past 27 years, few had pure kidney Yang deficiency. Modern life always causes energy blockage in certain parts of the body, such as the upper, middle and lower burners. We have to open up the channels so that we can bring the vital energy to the kidneys, spleen, liver, and testes. Furthermore, we consume more heat-producing foods than our parents' generation. Even if there is kidney Yang deficiency, we cannot simply tonify the kidney Yang.

The following are frequently used herbs to address kidney Yin deficiency, kidney Qi deficiency, blocked liver Qi, and weak digestive system. When we put a formula together, we need to balance Yin and Yang and also strengthen the digestive system. If a person cannot absorb the herbs, the formula cannot fully exert its effects.

> Huang Bai, Zhi Mu, Shu Di Huang, Shan Zhu Yu, Shan Yao, Rou Gui, Bai Zhu, Fu Ling, Chi Shao, Tu Si Zi, Chuan Niu Xi, Xian Mao

These herbs can tonify Yang and have sweet, acrid and warm properties. They can get into the liver and kidneys. Clinically, we use these herbs to treat infertility, ED, urinary problems and cold painful lower back and knees. Yin Yang Huo can also unblock Yang Qi flow in channels to treat arthritis, neck and lower back pain, muscle spasms, cramps, numbness, and other joint pain.

Two main chemicals in Yin Yang Huo, Icariin and Icaritin, are anti-inflammatory compounds. These can down-regulate tumor necrosis factor alpha (TNF-α) and thereby balance the immune system and reduce inflammation. The compounds can also down-regulate prostaglandin and nitric oxide and facilitate macrophage infiltration to the inflamed area. It is interesting that Yin Yang Huo has been used to enhance the production of progesterone in women with infertility. The fact that progesterone deficiency can influence the immune function and cause autoimmune problems may be coincident with the finding about the anti-inflammatory effect of Yin Yang Huo. More research has indicated that lack of progesterone can lead to an imbalance of immune function, infertility, and chronic inflammation. Menopause women can also benefit by taking a formula containing these herbs to help slow down the sudden decline of progesterone. Only taking this one single herb, however, can lead to other critical problems such as kidney Yin deficiency. Chinese formulas are usually multi-targeted. Taking a single herb for a long time can always lead to other problems.

Case Study

Chinese Herbs, Low Testosterone and ED

There are two kinds of hypogonadism: primary and secondary. Primary failure is caused by a problem in the testicles whereas secondary hypogonadism indicates a problem in the pituitary gland or hypothalamus. This part of the brain fails to signal the testicles to produce testosterone. The condition can be caused by several factors such as Kallmann's syndrome, pituitary disorders, or radiation therapy for a brain tumor. Other causes may include inflammatory diseases like tuberculosis, HIV/ AIDS and the use of certain medications. Being significantly overweight at any age can impact testosterone levels along with elevated estrogen level. Testosterone levels tend to decrease slowly with age. However, the rate of decrease may differ greatly. Medications for diabetes, high blood pressure and depression may lead to ED and low testosterone levels. High stress can cause low testosterone level. Statin can lower testosterone dramatically because it reduces the raw material for production of testosterone: cholesterol.

Chinese Herbs for Low Testosterone Levels

Chinese herbal medicine is an important part of traditional Chinese medicine. Each formula is a unique combination of different herbs targeting different organs. The king herb targets the primary issue, followed by the minister herbs that target secondary complaints or enhance the function of the king herb, and lastly, assistant herbs to reduce the side effects. The herbs are guided to specific body parts or channels for optimal results. Treatment with Chinese herbs and acupuncture helps to optimize your body's function. A study published in the journal of *Translational Andrology and Urology* in 2017 by Hao Li and colleagues explained why Chinese herbs could help improve ED and testosterone level. In animal models, they observed that some Chinese herbs could activate nitric oxide synthase (NOS)-cyclic guanosine monophosphate (cGMP) pathway, which could relax smooth muscles in penis and make the erection stronger, reduce the oxidative stress, lower the intracellular Ca^{2+} level and enhance the production of testosterone by improving the circulation to the testicles.

Chinese herbs are used in a unique way to regain the normalcy of your body. Please approach a TCM practitioner to discuss your issues, and get reinvigorated!

The horny goat (Yin Yang Huo) herb was found many years ago by a Chinese peasant to make goat extremely horny. Now many companies have been trying to make pills from this herb. However, taking only one single herb can make the body produce too much heat, causing other problems such as inflammation in your gut and respiratory system, and insomnia. Moreover, different genetic makeup will make people respond to the herbs differently. Some people can have very strong reaction to a small dose of the herbs and can develop insomnia. Other people need a higher dose in order to achieve the therapeutic effect. The herbal formulas usually combine 4 to over 10 different herbs to enhance the therapeutic effect and reduce the unwanted effect. If you developed ED due to low testosterone or too much stress or poor circulation to your testicles, please consult a well-trained herbalist to get the right formula so you can take the formula for 3 to 6 months and improve your overall functions rather than just get stronger erection temporarily. Herbal formula can tackle the root cause of ED: poor circulation to the pennies and inflammation in different parts of the body.

Mr. Lucus was diagnosed with type II diabetes 15 years ago. He loves sweets but he does not eat much. His blood sugar has never been too high. He usually goes to bed very late. While enjoying the quietness in late night his genius brain can function much better. He often feels hungry in the middle of the nights and eats some sweet food to make him happy. His blood A1c is usually between 6% to 6.8%. He has a lot of inflammation in his knees, hips and shoulders which he uses the most in his daily gardening work. He started taking herbs for his digestive issue many years ago because the Metformin he took for his diabetes blocked the digestion of carbs. With help of Chinese herbs his diarrhea has finally stopped, and, surprisingly, his ED has been improved. He had much stronger erections with the help of herbs and acupuncture. He is now 72 years old, and is still able to build a beautiful garden and lift heavy weight. His strong arm and leg muscles help maintain his testosterone level. Usually, the testosterone will gradually decline one percent every year after the age of 45 years old. Mr. Lucus has been physically active, which helps his blood circulation to his penis and testicles. If Mr. Lucus can go to bed earlier and avoid processed food, inflammation in his joints will be reduced and he would have higher level testosterone and less knee and shoulder pain. His positive attitude towards life may have contributed to his normal erection function too. With frequent smiling and laughing, your stress hormones are dropping and your body produces more happy hormones to fight the inflammation. Mr. Lucus loves tea with his sweets. Tea helps stabilize blood sugar and has anti-oxidative effect, and therefore can protect the blood vessels and nerves. On the other hand, drinking coffee can constrict blood vessels to your joints and eyes and also make your blood sugar drop too fast, which can make people crave for sweets even more.

Mr. Lucus also loves meditation when he takes a rest from his yard work. Combining meditation and acupuncture treatment, he can produce more nitric oxide (NO) gas and dilate the blood vessels to his hand, feet, eyes, testicles and pennies, which help him prevent ED in the future.

Part 2

Prostate Problems

Chapter 5

Prostate Enlargement and Elevated PSA

Prostate and its functions

The prostate is a walnut-sized gland that forms part of the male reproductive system. The gland is made of two parts enclosed by an outer layer of tissue. The prostate is located in front of the rectum and just below the bladder, where urine is stored. The prostate also surrounds the urethra, the canal through which urine passes out of the body. Not all of the prostate's functions are known. One of its main roles, though, is to squeeze fluid into the urethra as sperm moves through during sexual climax. This fluid, which helps make up semen, energizes the sperm and makes the vaginal canal less acidic. It is common for the prostate gland to become enlarged as a man ages. Doctors call this condition benign prostatic hyperplasia (BPH). In the United States in 2000, there were 4.5 million visits to physicians for prostatic enlargement. As a man matures, the prostate goes through two main periods of growth. The first occurs early in puberty, when the prostate doubles in size. At around age 25, the gland begins to grow again. The second growth phase often results, years later, in prostatic hyperplasia.

Though the prostate continues to grow during most of a man's life, the enlargement doesn't usually cause problems until late in life. Prostatic hyperplasia rarely causes symptoms before age 40, but more than half of men in their sixties and as many as 90% in their seventies and eighties have some symptoms of prostatic hyperplasia. As the prostate enlarges, the layer of tissue surrounding it stops it from expanding, causing the gland to press against the urethra like a clamp on a garden hose. The bladder wall becomes thicker and irritated. The bladder begins to contract even when it contains only small amounts of urine, causing more frequent urination. Eventually, the bladder weakens and loses the ability to empty itself, so that some of the urine remains in the bladder. The narrowing of the urethra and partial emptying of the bladder cause many of the problems associated with prostatic hyperplasia.

For many years, it has been known that prostatic hyperplasia occurs mainly in older men and that it doesn't develop in men whose testes were removed before puberty. For this reason, some researchers believe that factors related to aging and the testes may spur the development of prostatic hyperplasia. If removing the testes in puberty prevents prostate enlargement just because of the resulting low testosterone, then the decreasing testosterone associated with aging should not lead to enlargement of the prostate. There must be other factors involved in prostate enlargement in older men. I think the two growing periods of the prostate during puberty and the early twenties are closely related with later prostatic enlargement. Then why do some men not have urine problems while others have to get up to urinate every two hours during the night? Inflammation is the key factor here.

What is benign prostate hyperplasia?

Benign prostate hyperplasia (BPH) is the enlargement of the prostate gland, which occurs in 50% of men in their fifties and 90% of men in their eighties. Most men with BPH show the following symptoms: frequent and urgent urination, especially at night, slow urine flow, difficulty emptying the bladder, and urine dribbling. However, not every man with BPH has the above symptoms. Instead, inflammation and the balance of the nervous systems play an important role in how bad the urination problems can be. An 84-year-old man can still sleep through the night if he eats healthy, is active physically, and does not have inflammation in his prostate. On the other hand, a forty-year-old man who eats a lot of simple sugars and drinks one glass of wine every day may have high cholesterol with inflamed blood vessels and nerves and could get up three times at night. In order to reduce inflammation, we need eat a healthy diet and also keep our nervous and immune systems in balance. If you constantly stimulate your nerves with coffee or simple sugars, you may suffer from frequent urination and may not be able to hold your urine. Coffee can aggravate your urgency to urinate, while tea may help you hold the urine for a longer time.

What causes prostatic hyperplasia?

1.	Diabetes causes inflammation in the blood vessels and prostate: high blood sugar can lead to inflammation of the prostate and the capsule around the prostate. High blood sugar can also make your bladder more sensitive to the urine stored there.

2.	High estrogen: obesity and alcohol can lead to higher levels of estrogen, which stimulates prostate growth. More belly fat means more estrogen, less testosterone, and a bigger prostate. If a 25-year-old man has imbalanced estrogen and testosterone due to too much alcohol and sugar intake, the abnormal amounts of estrogen can cause overgrowth of the prostate during this period of time when the prostate naturally grows much faster than other times. If a young man already has a bigger than normal prostate, the prostate will exceed the normal size even more later with aging. That is why it is critical to control the abnormal growth of the prostate during this second, normal fast growth period. That is why people who drink too much alcohol or eat too much sugar at an early age will have more trouble holding their urine when they reach 40 or 50 years old.

3. Another theory focuses on dihydrotestosterone (DHT), a substance derived from testosterone in the prostate, which stimulates its growth. Some research has indicated that even with a drop in blood testosterone level, older men continue to produce and accumulate high levels of DHT in the prostate. This accumulation of DHT may encourage the growth of prostate cells. Scientists have also noted that men who do not produce DHT do not develop prostatic hyperplasia.

4. Regular alcohol consumption will compromise liver function, so estrogen cannot be deactivated after it has finished its job, resulting in high levels of estrogen and enlargement of prostate. Even one glass of wine a day can cause inflammation in the prostate, leading to prostate enlargement after age 40.

5. Spicy food produces a lot of heat inside your body, leading to inflammation in men's prostate and testes. Spicy food can also stimulate the peripheral nerves so your bladder is more sensitive to pressure and other stimulation.

6. Tensile strength of the prostate capsule: If the capsule outside the prostate loses its elasticity, the enlarged prostate cannot grow outward and instead will compress the urethra, causing more irritation. This is one of the reasons why the same amount of prostate enlargement can cause severe

urination problems in some men but not others with very stretchy prostate capsules. Lack of Vitamin C can cause this dysfunction of the prostate capsule. Drinking alcohol or smoking regularly will influence your digestive function such that minerals and vitamins cannot be absorbed effectively.

7.   Fish oil: A study published in *Journal of the National Cancer Institute* in 2013 showed the findings of researchers from the University of Washington, the National Cancer Institute, and Cleveland Clinic. They analyzed levels of Omega-3 fatty acids in the blood of 834 men who developed prostate cancer and race- and age-matched 1,393 men who did not develop prostate cancer. Men who had the highest levels of Omega-3 fatty acids had a 43% increase in risk for prostate cancer and 71% increase in risk for the high-grade prostate cancer that is the most likely to be fatal. Clinically, I have seen many cases of men, including body builders, who take very high dosage of fish oil, had elevated PSA for many years, and eventually developed prostate cancer. If you would like to have a higher level of Omega-3, maybe you should eat flax seeds, which have less concentrated Omega-3 combined with fiber. In that way, the Omega-3 will not be absorbed as fast as if you took fish oil. I have interviewed many healthy 90-year-old men in the past 10 years. They did not take fish oil. They just ate fish, chicken, and other whole grain foods. Once you take away the fiber, the absorption of Omega-3 becomes much faster.

What leads to prostatic hyperplasia symptoms?

Many symptoms of prostatic hyperplasia stem from obstruction of the urethra and a gradual loss of bladder function, which results in incomplete emptying of the bladder. The symptoms of prostatic hyperplasia vary, but the most common ones involve problems with urination, such as a hesitant, interrupted, and weak stream; urgency and leaking or dribbling; and more frequent urination, especially at night.

The size of the prostate does not always determine how severe the obstruction or the symptoms will be. Some men with greatly enlarged glands have little obstruction and few symptoms while others, whose glands are less enlarged, have more blockage and greater problems. This is associated with the bladder and urethra function and how sensitive your nerves are. If you already have compromised bladder function due to diabetes, neuropathy, or high blood pressure and you tend to have bladder and urethra inflammation, your symptoms may be more severe even with a slightly enlarged prostate. If men live long enough, almost everyone will develop prostate enlargement, but only 50% of men will have clinical symptoms. The above reason may explain why the other 50% have very limited urination problems. I have treated a 91-year-old gentleman, who still sleeps for 6 to 8 hours without getting up to urinate. I am sure at 91 years old, this gentleman has an enlarged prostate, but he has led such a healthy lifestyle that he does not have inflammation in his blood vessels, prostate, bladder and the nerves which control the bladder. Medication may also play a role in developing clinical symptoms.

Sometimes, a man may not know he has any obstruction until he suddenly finds himself unable to urinate at all. Taking over-the-counter cold or allergy medicines may trigger this condition called acute urinary retention. Such medicines contain decongestant drugs, also known as sympathomimetic drugs. A potential side effect of this kind of drugs may interrupt normal bladder and urethra function, causing the patient to be unable to urinate suddenly. When partial obstruction is present, alcohol, cold temperatures, or a long period of immobility also can bring on urinary retention. Urine retention and strain on the bladder can lead to urinary tract infections, bladder or kidney damage, bladder stones, incontinence, and the inability to control urination. If the bladder is permanently damaged, acupuncture treatment for prostatic hyperplasia may be ineffective. Therefore, when urine retention happens, getting immediate acupuncture treatment is very important to prevent permanent damage of the kidneys and bladder.

Chapter 6

How to use acupuncture and herbs to cope with BPH

How to prevent urination problems if prostatic hyperplasia is diagnosed

Apply heat to the lower abdominal area if the bladder cannot relax or contract normally.

Exercise the bladder muscles with Kegel exercises which may help prevent urine incontinence.

Moxa on CV4 (on the midline of the abdomen, 3 cun below the umbilicus), CV3 (on the midline of the abdomen, 4 cun below the umbilicus), KI5 (1 cun directly below KI3 in the depression between medial malleolus and tendon calcaneus, at the level of tip of medial malleolus).

Drink plenty of water to prevent bladder infection. Most men are worried about drinking water when a bathroom is not nearby. Men who drink more water do not necessarily go to bathroom more often than men who do not drink as much water. Additionally, the urgency can be reduced if a man drinks enough water. If you would like to relax your bladder muscles, you can drink more tea and less coffee or alcohol.

Cut down alcohol intake or stop completely if you already are diagnosed with BPH, especially if your PSA level keeps going up every year. This indicates that inflammation of the prostate may get worse and worse, which can change gene expression and eventually cause prostate cancer.

Use acupuncture or acupressure to strengthen the bladder muscles and regenerate the nerves that control the bladder muscles. Especially after prostate surgery, the sooner you have acupuncture, the less chance that you will develop ED or urine incontinence.

Avoid certain medications if you already experience difficulty urinating, such as cold medication. Do not hold your urine too long, which will over-stretch the bladder muscles.

Reduce coffee intake. Coffee is a diuretic and stimulates your nerves so you have more urgency to urinate. Coffee makes you run to the bathroom much more urgently/ frequently than does tea. Tea can relax your bladder muscles, but too much tea may also cause urine retention, kidney stones and bladder lining irritation.

Drinking dandelion herbal tea may help reduce the inflammation generally.

Eating a lot of fruits and vegetables, especially cruciferous vegetables such as kale, cauliflower, and cabbage will help reduce bad estrogen's stimulation of the prostate growth. Those vegetables can block the production of bad estrogen by blocking the aromatase enzyme.

Practice meditation to bring down estrogen levels. According to Dr. John Grey, PhD, when men are angry, they produce more estrogen. Moreover, anger can damage your immune function, leading to chronic inflammation in your body.

Taking Chinese herbs can not only enhance your testosterone production by improving the function of your endocrine system, but also reduce the inflammation of your prostate and lower your PSA level. Electro-acupuncture can also help strengthen your bladder muscle function, so you can sleep better and have a stronger immune function and a more balanced nervous system.

Research on acupuncture and BPH

The most popular medications in the treatment of BPH include α_1-andrenergic receptor blockers and 5α-reductase inhibitors, which relax the smooth muscles and reduce the size of the prostate (Rittmaster R.S. and Bartsch G., et. al. 2000, 2002). A newer type of medication, namely phosphodiesterase type 5 (PDE5) inhibitors, can also reduce the symptoms of BPH (Oelke M. et. al 2013). These medications, however, do not target the root cause of BPH: inflammation and imbalance of cell growth and death. Long term use of these medications can cause blood loss, urinary incontinence, infection, sexual dysfunction, and morphological changes in the prostate (Kyprianou N. 2003). If the inflammation continues for more than 10 years, the level of PSA will rise. Once the level of PSA goes beyond 10, the possibility of prostate cancer will increase. Therefore, it is critical to use acupuncture and herbs to get rid of the inflammation in the prostate and restore the balance of the hormones; otherwise, these men will have to use medications forever. Notably, more and more younger men are suffering ED nowadays. Finding safer treatments can help them prevent ED in the future.

The normal function and size of the prostate is regulated through a delicate balance of cell death and proliferation. If old cells cannot be cleared up through programmed cell death called apoptosis, then the prostate will grow bigger and bigger. Recent research indicates that hormone imbalance plays an important role in BPH. For example, the imbalance of testosterone and estrogen can affect the synthesis of certain enzymes and chemicals, which leads to inflammation and the reduction of programmed cell death. Chughtai and colleagues demonstrated that nitric oxide synthetase can activate reactive nitrogen which is able to damage prostate cells (Chughtai et al. 2011). In hyperplastic prostate tissue, the synthesis of nitric oxide is higher than in normal tissues (Wang et al. 2011). Suar and his colleagues observed that nitric oxide could be converted by cox enzymes to prostaglandins in the epithelium and interstitial space of inflammatory cells of the prostate. Prostaglandins are known to induce inflammation.

The findings by S. Sahin et al. published in *Prostate Cancer and Prostatic Diseases* in 2015 have proven that acupuncture can help reduce urine problems. One hundred patients with chronic prostatitis and chronic pelvic pain syndrome were randomized to receive acupuncture at either seven standard acupoints bilaterally or sham points adjacent to these points. A National Institutes of Health Chronic Prostatitis Symptom Index was completed by each patient before and 6, 8, 16, and 24 weeks after the treatment. The higher score the patient had, the more severe their symptoms were. The results showed that the use of acupuncture in the treatment of men with chronic prostatitis/chronic pelvic pain syndrome resulted in a significant decrease in total Chronic

Prostatitis Symptom Index scores, indicating significant relief of the clinical symptoms.

In a research conducted by Dr. Y.Y. Pen et al., 200 patients with benign prostate enlargement were recruited and randomized into an acupuncture only group and an acupuncture plus moxibustion group. Each group had 100 patients. Acupuncture stimulation was applied on the point UB54 with triple filiform needles. Other main acupuncture points, such as Pang-Shuidao (one cun beside ST28); Pang-Guilai (one cun beside ST29); Shenshu (BL23); Sanyinjiao (SP6); Guanyuan (CV4); Zhongji (CV3), and some supplemental acupuncture points selected according to each person's individual symptoms, were also stimulated with filiform needles. The acupuncture plus moxibustion group was also treated with bird-pecking moxibustion on UB54 and moxa stick segments attached to needles for the other acupuncture points. Two groups were treated for 30 min, 3 times a week. Patients were evaluated before and after the treatments. The International Prostate Symptom Scores (IPSS) of the two groups were significantly decreased compared with pre-treatment scores in the same group (P<0.01). The acupuncture only group had 23% and the acupuncture with moxibustion had 42% of patients achieving remarkable improvement of the urinary problems.

Interestingly, 26% of the acupuncture group had no improvement while only 11% of acupuncture plus moxibustion group had no improvement of the urinary symptoms. The effective rates were 74% for the acupuncture only group and 89% for the acupuncture plus moxibustion group.

In conclusion, if the acupuncturist can teach patients to do moxibustion at home every day and get acupuncture treatment twice or three times a week for 12 to 24 weeks, the effective rate for treating prostate enlargement-related symptoms will be much higher than just getting acupuncture once a week. Furthermore, patients can achieve stronger erections and deeper sleep when all the urination problems are gone with acupuncture treatments.

Dr. Xu conducted another clinical study comparing acupuncture-moxibustion and herbal treatment for patients with BPH, and the results were published in *Zhong Guo Zhen Jiu* in 2014. One hundred and twenty-eight patients were randomized into an acupuncture-moxibustion group and a Qianliekang (a Chinese herbal formula for enlarged prostate) group with 64 people in each group. In the acupuncture-moxibustion group, acupuncture was applied to Shenshu (BL23), Pangguangshu (BL28), Zhongji (CV3), Guanyuan

(CV4), and Shuidao (ST28), and the warm moxibustion therapy with moxa sticks was used at Shenshu (BL 23), Guanyuan (CV4) and Shenque (CV8) once every day. In the Qianliekang group, Qianliekang tablets were prescribed for oral administration, 4 tablets each time, three times a day for 3 months. The IPSS and the changes in residual urine (RU) and maximum urine flow rate (Qmax) determined with the ultrasonic B test were compared before and after treatment in the two groups. The results of the IPSS, maximum urine flow rate, and residual urine improved dramatically after treatment as compared to before treatment in the two groups. The improvements in the acupuncture-moxibustion group were much more obvious than those in the herbal tablet group. The total effective rate was 89.1% in the acupuncture-moxibustion group, which was better than the 68.7% effective rate in the herbal tablet group.

Ricci et al. found that electro-acupuncture had better effects in decreasing the number of urination and urinary urgency that persisted after transurethral resection of the prostate. Clinically, most men who do not receive acupuncture treatment after prostate surgery use the bathroom 2-3 times more at night than those who receive acupuncture treatment after surgery.

Philip et al. observed that acupuncture can increase bladder capacity in patients with bladder instability. Especially when a man holds more than 300 cc of urine after he empties his bladder, acupuncture has been clinically proven to reduce the residual urine. Most men can sleep better after their acupuncture treatment. Acupuncture treatment has an accumulating effect.

Yang Wang et al. added further evidence to the use of acupuncture for patients with BPH. Their research indicated that the IPSS was decreased by 7.26 in the acupuncture group with the stimulation on BL33, compared to 2.34 decreases in the non-point electro-acupuncture group. This study also demonstrates that sacral neuromodulation can improve symptoms of an overactive bladder, so the urgency and frequency of the urination are reduced. Furthermore, acupuncture has a better effect than that of terazosin. Also, in their pilot trial, 40 patients were randomized into the treatment group (BL33) and the control group (non-point acupuncture site located beside BL33). The results show that electro-acupuncture at BL33 has a better effect not only in reducing IPSS and bladder residual urine, but also increases the maximum urinary flow rate more than electro-acupuncture at a non-point.

When men reach 50 years of age, about 50% of them experience frequent night urination, urgency to urinate, and urine retention. These symptoms can influence their sleep and social life, creating anxiety and insomnia. Medications can help relax the smooth muscles of the bladder and the prostate to reduce the urgency and frequency of urination but can also lead to ED and urine retention.

Observations by Qin et al. about using acupuncture to treat chronic prostatitis and chronic pelvic pain syndrome were published in 2018 in the *Journal of Urology*. This research was a 32-week randomized controlled trial, which included 8 weeks of treatment and then 24 weeks of follow-up. Sixty-eight patients ranging from 18 to 50 years old were randomly assigned to acupuncture or non-invasive sham acupuncture. The National Institutes of Health Chronic Prostatitis Symptom Index (NIH-CPSI) total scores differed significantly between the two groups at 8, 20, and 32 weeks after treatment. There were no significant differences between the groups in NIH-CPSI pain and quality of life subscale scores and IPSS at week 4 (p>0.05 for all). For all other secondary outcomes, the acupuncture group was statistically better than the sham acupuncture group. The researchers concluded that acupuncture showed clinical and long-lasting benefits compared with sham acupuncture for chronic prostatitis and chronic pelvic pain syndrome, but a sufficient dosage was needed to achieve the best result.

Interestingly, electro-acupuncture can reduce the symptoms of chronic prostatitis but does not reduce the level of testosterone. These benefits may be related to improved testicular function due to electro-acupuncture on points of the kidney and bladder meridians.

If men do not have time to do acupuncture treatments twice a week for 8 weeks, they may be able to use saline or herbal injections to reduce the frequency of the acupuncture treatment needed. The following study supports this interesting combination of electro-acupuncture and point injection for prostate enlargement.

A research article written by K.M. Seong et al. titled "Hwanglyunhaedok Pharmacopuncture versus Saline Pharmacopuncture on Chronic Nonbacterial Prostatitis/ Chronic Pelvic Pain Syndrome" was published in the *Journal of Acupuncture Meridian Studies* in 2017. In this study, 63 patients diagnosed with chronic prostatitis/chronic pelvic pain syndrome was treated with electro-acupuncture and 8 injections of 1 mL of herbal solution or saline at the acupoint CV1 twice a week for 4 weeks. The herbal injection group had 32 patients, and the saline group had 31 patients. After twice a week treatment for 4 weeks, researchers found that the total NIH-CPSI scores were significantly reduced in both groups. Pain scores in both groups also decreased significantly. In addition, IPSS reduced significantly after treatment in both groups. There was no significant difference between the herbal injection and saline injection groups in NIH-CPSI scores and IPSS.

Electro-acupuncture can reduce the symptoms of BPH but not the level of testosterone. This has been verified by R. Zheng in 2017 as published in the journal *Zhong Guo Zhen Jiu*. Sixty patients were randomized into an electro-acupuncture group and a medication group with 30 people in each one. In the electro-acupuncture group, electro-acupuncture was applied to the points Zhongji (CV3) and Qugu (CV2), once a day, 5 times a week. In the medication group, 0.2 mg of tamsulosin hydrochloride sustained-release capsules were prescribed for oral administration once a day. The duration of treatment was 6 weeks in both groups. Changes in serum testosterone (T), estradiol (E_2), E_2/T, IPSS, erectile function score (II EF5), serum PSA, and adverse reactions were observed before and after treatment in the two groups. Clinical therapeutic effects were compared between the two groups. The differences in serum T, E_2, and E_2/T

were not significant in the electro-acupuncture group (all $P>0.05$) before and after treatment, but the difference in E_2/T was significant in the medication group ($P<0.05$). IPSS was reduced after electro-acupuncture treatment ($P<0.05$) but was not significantly reduced after treatment with medication ($P>0.05$). The difference after treatment was significant ($P<0.05$) between the two groups, with the electro-acupuncture group having better effects. After treatment, symptom severity was noticeably reduced in the electro-acupuncture group, and the patients' overall situation was better than that of the medication group ($P<0.05$). The total effective rate was 60.7% in the electro-acupuncture group, almost doubled the improvement rate of 30.8% ($P<0.05$) in the medication group. This study indicates that electro-acupuncture can relieve the symptoms of chronic prostatitis more efficiently without changing serum testosterone and estrogen levels very much.

Treating BPH with herbs

In 2017, Dr. S.J. Shin published an article about how a traditional Korean herbal formula suppresses testosterone-induced BPH by regulating inflammatory responses and programmed cell death (apoptosis) in rats in the journal *Experimental and Therapeutic Medicine*. In this study, researchers applied testosterone for 4 weeks to induce BPH in the rats. Then, they gave the Korean herbal formula to the rats for 4 weeks. Changes in prostate weight, testosterone, and DHT levels were compared to those of the rats without the herbal formula treatment. Cyclooxygenase-2 (Cox-2) and inducible nitric oxide synthase (iNOS) played important roles in the inflammation of the prostate tissue. The levels of COX-2 and iNOS proteins in the BPH group were higher than those in the control group. In contrast, COX-2 and iNOS levels in the Korean herb group were lower than those in the BPH group without the herbs. The decrease in COX-2 and iNOS in the group with Korean herbs indicated that the inflammation in the prostate was reduced.

Chapter 7

Acupuncture and BPH Case Studies

Case 1: Stronger erections with acupuncture treatments after prostate removal

Larry Lee had prostate cancer surgery in 1997 at the age of 58. After surgery, his PSA levels were within normal range, indicating no further prostate issues. He was a slightly over-weighted man with high levels of cholesterol, for which he had been treated with Lipitor during the previous 5 years. He came to see me eight years after his surgery, complaining that his erections did not last as long as before the surgery. Also, he complained of pain in his right elbow. As we spoke further, he told me that in the morning, when his bladder was full, his erection was strong and lasted a long time. He used to have very satisfying sex with his wife. After the surgery, he had impotence for a year. His erection gradually came back, but not as strong as before. His penis sensation also changed; the entire tip of his penis used to be very sensitive, but now only the top part had some sensation and felt dry during intercourse. Therefore, it became more difficult to achieve orgasm with the same amount of stimulation.

At the age of 66, sexual function will naturally decrease, especially if men do not take care of their health. When the prostate is removed, fluid secretion will decrease. Larry Lee could achieve very solid erections, but once his penis entered a dry vagina, he would lose his erection. He tried Viagra, which gave him a super strong erection, but because he has high blood pressure and high cholesterol, he worried about strokes and heart problems. Every time he came to see me, I measured his blood pressure, which was around 150/85 mmHg. He had some nerve damage around his surgery area with a scar line from 1 inch to 3 inches below his belly button, which contributed to his sensory loss. But he could still get a good erection and strong orgasm through masturbation, indicating the blood flow to his penis and the nerves responsible for his erection were still pretty good. His wife had had a hysterectomy, resulting in extreme vaginal dryness that led to painful intercourse. When he saw his wife in pain, he quickly lost his erection. In this regard, his sexual function was almost normal for his age. I recommended that his wife use bioidentical estrogen cream to help the vaginal dryness.

When he first came to see me, his PSA had started creeping up, and he had urgency to urinate and partial incontinence. I tried to strengthen his kidney and bladder function by tonifying the points KI5 (1 cun directly below KI3 in the depression anterior and superior to the medial side of the tuberosity of the calcaneum), KI7 (2 cun directly above KI3 on the anterior border of tendon-calcaneus), and CV4 (on the midline of the abdomen, 3 cun below the umbilicus). In the meantime, I tried to clear his heat due to kidney Yin deficiency and invigorate his blood flow so that his PSA could get back to normal. After 4 treatments, he noticed that his morning erection lasted a longer time. Even after he emptied his bladder, he could get another spontaneous erection for a good amount of time. After 5 more treatments, he had much more control of his urination. Surprisingly, when he went on a trip, he could have intercourse with his wife with great satisfaction. However, if he or his wife became tired or stressed out, vaginal intercourse became difficult.

Larry Lee had slightly elevated blood pressure, especially when his stress level was high, but he was not taking any medications for his high blood pressure. I was surprised that his physician never gave him medication for his high blood pressure. Maybe this was one of the reasons why he was able to get his sexual function back after prostate surgery, since blood pressure medications can lead to impotence.

After 24 acupuncture treatments once or twice a week, Larry Lee had no urinary incontinence. His urine flow became stronger. He only needed to get up once during the night to go to the bathroom and he was able to fall back to sleep right away. Larry Lee always came for his acupuncture treatment before a vacation with his wife and reported that he would have wonderful sex during each trip. His elbow pain also went away with acupuncture. However, his blood pressure still fluctuated depending on how stressful his day was. Surprisingly, he never had dizziness, neck stiffness, or bad temper with his blood pressure fluctuating between 150/95 and 120/80 mmHg.

Case 2: Relapse of prostate cancer with increased PSA

John Prevaza was born in Weston and went to Boston College to study engineering. He had been trained as a hard worker and loved to drink beer to help him relax during his four years of college. After graduation, he worked for a company in Needham and continued drinking 2 to 3 beers every night at home. He also loved soda, and his belly gradually grew with a lot of fat tissue accumulating around the internal organs.

When he first came to Boston Chinese Acupuncture, he had already finished surgery for prostate removal at Newton

Wellesley Hospital. His PSA dropped from 20 to 0.2 after the surgery. After reading some information about acupuncture and prostate cancer written by one of the acupuncturists in the Boston area, he wanted to strengthen his immunity and bladder function because his urination at night had become so frequent that he had to get up more than 3 times each night, which interrupted his deep sleep and made him very tired during the day. Sometimes, he could not find the restroom right away, and he started to develop urinary incontinence. He was planning to retire soon, but he needed to solve the urinary problems while he was still working at his company and had their insurance coverage.

His acupuncturist told him that even though his PSA was very low, there were still some cancer cells floating in his body. He really needed to stop or cut down his alcohol intake to prevent prostate cancer from coming back. He said beer really helped him relax after his hard work at his company. After coming to acupuncture treatment once a week for a few months, his bladder and kidney functions became stronger. He also cut down his beer to once or twice a week during the treatment, and his PSA stayed below 2 for a few years.

He retired and moved to downtown Boston and enjoyed walking near Boston Harbor. At this point, he came for acupuncture treatment every two weeks. He started travelling with his girlfriend while driving his trailer around different states in the U.S. While travelling, he started increasing his beer intake. When he came back to have acupuncture treatment one year after his retirement, his PSA had increased from 0.2 to 10. His urologist told him that the prostate cancer had come back and that he had to take Lupron to block testosterone. A few weeks after he started hormone treatment, he began to have hot flushes and night sweats. He felt so miserable that he decided to stop his beer intake and instead drink herbal tea. With acupuncture treatment twice a week for 5 months at Boston Chinese Acupuncture, his hot flushes and night sweats became under control. His PSA dropped from 10 to 5. The acupuncturist recommended a diet with more cruciferous vegetables to block the conversion of the testosterone into estrogen. He started eating kale, cooked cauliflower, brussel sprouts, and broccoli. Initially, he could not digest those anti-cancer vegetables, so he had to start with a small amount. After a few months, he found that his PSA dropped to below 5 and no longer needed to use Lupron to block his testosterone. He was then almost 70 years old, and the prostate cancer had gone into remission. However, the Lupron caused muscle loss, and his impotence came back.

According to research by Dr. M.C. Bosland of the University of Illinois at Chicago, prostate cancer incidence was markedly increased when estradiol was applied to lab rats for a short period of time. The mechanism is that too much estrogen can damage DNA and stimulate tumor-cell activators. One of the reasons why men can develop breast cancer if they consume too much fat, sugar, or alcohol is because of the abnormal level of bad estrogen.

Case 3: Diabetic neuropathy with enlarged prostate

Don Levi is a 76-year-old retired engineer. He reported an episode of cystitis (inflamed bladder) at least 30 years ago, at which time he also had incomplete bladder emptying. He was diagnosed with type II diabetes, colitis, hypertension, and high cholesterol in his early forties. Part of his thyroid was removed right after all of these problems were diagnosed. He never smoked or consumed alcohol, but since childhood, he ate a lot of sweets and a hot dog every day. At the age of 75, his PSA was 0.9 with residual urine in his bladder.

He was diagnosed with benign prostate enlargement in 2006. A couple of months after the diagnosis, he had laser ablation from the bladder neck to the center of the prostate, where the ejaculatory duct joins the urethra. According to his urologist's report, the surgery was very successful; a wide channel of his urethra was obtained. After such a procedure, a couple of weeks of discomfort is normal, with blood in the urine, extremely frequent urination, and a burning sensation at the tip of the penis. You would think his problems had been fixed, but three months after the surgery he came to my office. His complaints were frequent urination, urgency to urinate, unable to hold urine, slow and hesitant flow, diminished libido, and poor-quality erections, the exact same complaints he had before the surgery. He also had cataracts, depression, and anxiety. He urinated at night one or two times, with daytime frequency every 3 hours.

I carefully asked him about his urination. He woke up after 4 to 6 hours of sleep: the first time, he had difficulty initiating urination and his flow was very slow; the second time, one or two hours after the first urination, the urine flow became stronger. After 5 acupuncture treatments, his frequency of night urination was reduced to every 6 hours, and his urine flow became stronger for 3 days after his acupuncture treatment. His urination varied: sometimes better, other times worse. When his bladder was very full, he had difficulty getting urine out. Sometimes, he had to manipulate his penis with his hand to get urine out. He also noticed that when he drank more water, his urine flow seemed stronger. He was taking many medications: Asacol for colitis, Avandia for diabetes, Norvasc for hypertension, Levoxyl for low thyroid function, Lipitor for cholesterol, Atenelol for his heart, Tricor for triglycerides, Flomax for his prostate, and aspirin for his heart. Additionally, he took food supplements, including calcium-magnesium, chromium, Co-Enzyme Q10, ginseng, EPA, evening primrose, eye bright, glucosamine, Condroitin, lecithin, lutein, multi-vitamin, potassium, Prilosec, and vitamin C.

I was amazed at his ability to remember to take all these medications and supplements. I am sure my stomach and liver would not have been able to process all of those food supplements. I suggested that he talk to a dietician. He cut out potassium, vitamin c, lecithin, and lutein. Lecithin is a fatlike substance that helps increase the stool excretion of neutral steroid molecules. This may reduce the absorption of dietary cholesterol from the intestinal contents while restricting the reabsorption of endogenously produced cholesterol into the bloodstream. However, lecithin is in wheat, soybean, peanuts, maize, liver, oats, rice, trout, meat, eggs, and butter. As a diabetes patient, he had no problem taking whole wheat, soybean, and peanuts. His dietician told him that if he was unable to eat foods that are rich in certain nutrients or if he needed extra supplements (deficiency symptoms), then he should take certain food supplements. I usually tell my patients that if you do not have an illness and your digestive system is functioning, it is better to have whole foods than food supplements. If you are really worried about a lack of certain vitamins or minerals, take food supplements twice a week for long-term use or take them every day for a couple of months and then change to once a week. A recent study about vitamins indicated that most vitamins can be harmful if people take too much.

I treated Don Levi for 3 months with acupuncture and moxa. I told him that because he had diabetes, high blood pressure, and thyroid problems, the nerves controlling the bladder muscle and the muscle itself might have some inflammation. In order to strengthen the bladder muscle, he could try moxa and certain exercises. His blood sugar level could go up to 200 mg/dL two hours after eating, which could further damage his nerve function, so he had to find a way to lower his sugar level. After 12 treatments, his urine flow generally improved, with no dribbling at the end of urination. He did not have to rush to the bathroom after his hour long acupuncture treatment. He also noticed that his incontinence was gone, and he had stronger urine flow. He found out that grape juice seemed to increase his urine frequency and slow down urine flow. Interestingly, if he thought too much about his problems, his urine flow would become slower. At the end of 12 treatments, his spontaneous erections were more frequent at night, meaning the nerve function was improving. He stopped acupuncture treatments.

Six months after his laser surgery, Don Levi went back to his urologist for a routine checkup. His bladder was enlarged, and residual urine was about 800 cc, similar to his condition right after the surgery. This verified that the bladder muscle and nerves were damaged by high blood sugar. When the urologist examined his urethra, there was scar tissue build up due to the laser surgery 6 months earlier. Acupuncture helped reduce the bladder inflammation and strengthen the muscle, but the scar tissue blocked urine flow, so he could not empty his bladder effectively. His urologist suggested another surgery to remove the scar tissue. Don Levi was initially reluctant, but he eventually decided to have the second surgery to remove the scar tissue from the first laser surgery. Then, he was told to put a catheter in every day to prevent the urethra opening from closing and the scar tissue from building up. After surgery, he discharged a lot of blood clots in the urine, but he put the catheter into his urethra every day. His urine flow seemed to become stronger. One month after the surgery, he had a urinary tract infection and was rushed to the emergency room. Three months after the second surgery, Don Levi stopped using a catheter. His urine flow was not as strong as before, with still about 400 mL of urine left after each urination. His urologist told him that at this age, 400 mL of residual urine was normal.

To summarize, if he did not have the first laser surgery, the scar tissue would not have built up. He really needed to control his blood sugar level. I think the second surgery was necessary, but finding out the reason for the bladder muscle and nerve problems was the key factor in avoiding further damage.

Case 4: Prostate cancer, ED, and aneurysm

Mr. Li came to Boston Chinese Acupuncture for his left ankle pain in 2016. He had been practicing Taekwondo for many years and had multiple injuries around his ankles. His right knee had a partial replacement, and his left ankle had a tendon transplant from a cadaver. It was amazing that he had no knee pain or swelling after his knee surgery. He said that he loved to eat sweets since childhood, and he was in the sugar business until he reached fifty years of age. He was a very smart man and made enough money that he could stop working in his early 50s. He loved travelling and collecting art work. It seemed that his life was perfect after retirement, with enough money and a beautiful wife.

He continued to eat small amount of sweets and drink about one glass of wine or other kind of alcohol every day. Ten years after retirement, he was diagnosed with prostate cancer. He had surgery to remove the prostate, using the newest, minimally invasive techniques at Boston Medical Center. His PSA came back to normal, and he was told he was free of cancer after that. However, after surgery, he felt numb in the lower abdominal area and developed impotence. He reported that he still had a strong sexual drive but he had developed ED and lost his morning erection, indicating that he suffered nerve damage after the prostate surgery. We used electro-acupuncture for 3 months to stimulate nerve regeneration and relieve his left ankle pain. Most of my patients can gain back their normal sexual function after 3 to 10 months of acupuncture treatment. Mr. Li had reduced ankle pain after 12 treatments and he was able to walk for 30 minutes without pain. Nevertheless, he continued to eat sweets and drink alcohol. Those two factors unfortunately could lead to inflammation of the nerves and blood vessels. He also had had diverticulitis (inflammation of the intestines) for many years. His digestion was not strong enough to absorb sufficient vitamins and minerals. Without these important nutrients, he could not repair the pelvic nerve and blood vessel damage as fast as other men who do not drink alcohol regularly and eat sweets every day after surgery. He was very patient in waiting for his nerves to regenerate so that he could restore his functions.

A few months after I treated Mr. Li, he got his blood work done, and his testosterone was 500 ng/dL, which was not bad for a 75-year-old. In the meantime, he was told that he had an aneurysm in his lower abdominal area, which could cause severe bleeding. This is another sign of inflammation in his blood vessels, which causes the weakening of the blood vessels due to diet and digestive problems. He had surgery to remove the aneurysm in the fall of 2017 at Newton Wellesley Hospital and he recovered well with regular acupuncture treatments. His ED was not yet fixed because of his diet. Mr. Li has been very patient, but he needs to change his diet and improve his absorption of vitamins and minerals in order to regenerate his nerves in the perineum area.

When we pass a certain age, our growth hormones and testosterone are much lower than people in their twenties. It will take a longer time for us to recover from any trauma. Prostate surgery does damage to some nerves that control erections. It is very critical to improve circulation so that the nerves can regenerate.

How to use Chinese herbs and acupuncture to optimize your PSA level

Elevated PSA indicates inflammation in your prostate. When men reach 80 years of age, most of them will have an enlarged prostate. If prostate inflammation is under control, they will have fewer symptoms such as urgency to urinate, slow flow and frequent urination. When a man has to get up 2 to 3 times at night, his deep sleep will be interrupted. His body and mind cannot rejuvenate, and he may quickly lose memory, develop arthritis, have a decreased testosterone level, and lose muscle mass and hair.

Doing the following may help optimize your PSA level

Cut down your coffee intake. Coffee stimulates the sympathetic nervous system, causing urgency of urination. When your nervous system is hyperactive, your immune function will be out of balance, which can lead to chronic inflammation. Also, you tend to urinate more frequently than people who drink tea or just water. You can drink dandelion and honeysuckle tea to clear up the inflammation.

Eliminate or reduce alcohol intake. Generally speaking, healthy 100-year-olds do not often drink alcohol. If they do, they drink very little. Alcohol produces a lot of internal heat, which can cause inflammation in the nerves and prostate. In addition, alcohol can make men produce higher levels of estrogen, which stimulates the prostate to grow bigger and develop more inflammation.

Cut down on processed food. The purified sugar leads to inflammation in your prostate and in other parts of your body.

Practice acupressure on the abdominal area so that you can improve the circulation to your prostate and clear up the inflammatory chemicals. Having acupuncture treatment once or twice a week for 6 months can clear the heat and reduce the inflammation. Taking Chinese herbs helps reduce inflammation and the urgency of urination. Chinese herbs can also help you optimize your testosterone levels.

Case 5: Chinese herbs, fish oil, and PSA

Mr. Lin came to Boston for his post-doctoral study when he was 30 years old. He had been busy with his studies and really enjoyed coffee and soda because those drinks are cheap and convenient. After Mr. Lin finished his post-doctoral training at Boston College, he found a job as a research scientist at a biotech company. He was so passionate about his research project that he did not have time to cook or buy healthy food.

When Mr. Lin turned 40 years old, he noticed that his sleep pattern had changed. He had to get up 2 to 3 times at night to go to the bathroom. Mr. Lin had been a very good sleeper since his childhood. The interrupted sleep made him feel tired during the day, and he could not work as efficiently as he did before. He went to see his urologist at Newton Wellesley Hospital to figure out what was causing his frequent night urination. His urologist told him that his prostate was enlarged and was pressing on and irritating his bladder. His PSA was elevated to 4 ng/mL. Elevated PSA meant that he might have inflammation in his prostate.

As a researcher, he wanted to know what caused his PSA to go up and how he could lower it without medication. He did research on the internet and was very happy to find that fish oil could help an enlarged prostate. He immediately bought the most expensive fish oil from a vitamin store in downtown Boston. After Mr. Lin took fish oil for about 6 months, he went back to Newton Wellesley hospital for a PSA recheck. Surprisingly, his PSA had risen to 6 ng/mL. He also noticed that the frequency of his night urination had not been reduced, and his bladder seemed to have more residual urine. He was worried about his PSA because if it continued to go up, then there was a higher probability of developing prostate cancer. He came to Boston Chinese Acupuncture in Needham, hoping the acupuncturist and herbalist could help him normalize his PSA and reduce the frequency of night urination.

The acupuncturist asked about his diet and lifestyle and recommended that he get rid of processed foods and sugary drinks so that he can reduce his belly fat and estrogen. Then, he started acupuncture treatments twice a week for 6 weeks and then once a week for a year to reduce the inflammation in his prostate. Also, he started taking Chinese herbs to clear up the internal heat in his body. He lost 20 lbs. within 6 months. He went back to the hospital to get his PSA checked again, and was happy to know that his PSA dropped to 3 ng/mL. Now, Mr. Lin continues with acupuncture once a week to strengthen his kidney and bladder function. He is able to sleep through the night with improved memory and creative thinking. He was promoted to senior research scientist after he published a breakthrough research paper in *Science*.

Case 6: Acupuncture and Prostatitis

Larry is a 42-year-old businessman with two healthy children and a very stable and lucrative job in a finance company. When he was studying at Harvard Business School, he attended many drinking parties to connect with alumni so that he could find a job right after graduation. Business school parties always included alcohol. He was fortunate not to have any problems until he reached 35 years old. At that time, he started having pressure and a burning sensation in his lower abdominal area. Even sitting could cause pain. His lower back also started bothering him. His job in finance involved working in front of a computer, which made his symptoms even worse. He understood that he could not enjoy his luxurious lifestyle if he had poor health, so he went to Boston Medical Center to get his bladder, kidney, and prostate checked. Surprisingly, his prostate was not enlarged, and his PSA was within the normal range. His urologist at Boston Medical Center gave him medication to reduce the pressure and burning sensation in his lower abdominal area, and his condition quickly improved. He then continued with his wine and beer intake 7 days a week to reduce his stress after work.

After a year, this magic pill did not work anymore. Larry's pressure sensation came back, along with frequent night-time urination, even though his PSA remained within the normal range. Without sufficient sleep, he also started to experience foot and shoulder pain. Interestingly, his foot pain was located around the KI2 point of the kidney meridian, which is supposed to be related to urination and sexual function. He changed urologists and was told that he could try another medication. Although he faithfully started the new medication, it did not have any effect. Every day when he went to work, he hated sitting in front of his computer, and his attention span was not as long as before. Also, his memory started changing. His boss noticed that his performance was not as efficient as before in his small financial company in Boston. He was afraid to lose his job and decided to find a holistic practitioner in Needham, where his big house and beautiful yard are located. He could not afford to lose his job.

The acupuncturist at Boston Chinese Acupuncture examined Larry's tongue and pulse and suggested that he might have developed inflammation in his prostate even though his prostate was not enlarged. Such inflammation will sensitize the pelvic nerves and cause the pressure and burning sensation that he was experiencing. She recommended acupuncture twice a week for 12 weeks and then once a week for 12 more weeks. She also recommended that he cut down his alcohol consumption to twice or once a week. In this way, he could still enjoy alcohol without sacrificing his health. Changing habits is very stressful but suffering pressure and burning sensations is more stressful.

In order to relax after work, Larry started to substitute herbal tea for alcohol. Usually he arrived home around 6 PM, had dinner, and started drinking dandelion herbal tea. He also arranged to have twice-a-week acupuncture treatment for 6 weeks. His pressure sensation went away after 8 treatments. Surprisingly, he felt very happy after each treatment even though he stopped drinking alcohol. However, he noticed that he still had to wake up to go to the bathroom around 3 to 4 AM. His acupuncturist recommended that he drink his herbal tea right after work, at least 30 min before dinner. Then, he could enjoy a delicious dinner with his wife and children. The herbal tea helped him clear up the inflammation and reduce his daily stress. Now, he can sleep through the night and has better memory and more motivation.

During the treatment for his prostate inflammation, Larry's acupuncturist inserted needles into his KI2 point and his shoulder area. Then, his foot pain went away, and his shoulder pain stopped bothering him. He started playing golf with his business partners. By the time he finished 24 acupuncture treatments, he got promoted in his company because every day, he went to work with a big smile on his face, and his work efficiency increased, along with good relationships with his colleagues.

Bibliography

Bartsch, G., Rittmaster, R.S., and Klocker, H.
Dihydrotestosterone and the concept of 5alpha-reductase
inhibition in human benign prostatic hyperplasia. *Eur.
Urol.* 2000. 37:367-380.

Bartsch, G., Rittmaster, R.S., and Klocker, H.
Dihydrotestosterone and the concept of 5alpha-reductase
inhibition in human benign prostatic hyperplasia. *World J.
Urol.* 2002. 19:413-425.

Cakmak, H., Kocatürk, T., Dündar, S.O., et al. The Relationship
between Neovascular Age-Related Macular Degeneration
and Erectile Dysfunction. *J. Ophthalmology.* 2013.
10:1155. doi: 10.1155/2013/589274.

Chen, J.K. and Chen T. *Chinese Medical Herbology and
Pharmacology.* Art of Medicine Press. 2003. 894-895.

Chughtai, B., Lee, R., Te, A., et al. Role of inflammation in
benign prostatic hyperplasia. *Rev. Urol.* 2011.13:147-150.

Costa, C., and Virag, R. The endothelial-erectile dysfunction
connection: an essential update. *J. Sex Med.* 2009.
6:2390-2404. doi: 10.1111/j.1743-6109.2009.01356.x.

Cui X., Li X., Peng W., et al. Acupuncture for erectile dysfunction: a systematic review protocol. *BMJ. open* 2015. 5:e007040. 10.1136/bmjopen-2014-007040.

Cui, X., Zhou J., Qin Z., et al. Acupuncture for erectile dysfunction: a systematic review. *BioMed Research International*. 2016. 2016:2171923. doi: 10.1155/2016/2171923.

Fibbi, B., Penna, G., Morelli, A., et al. Chronic inflammation in the pathogenesis of benign prostatic hyperplasia. *Int. J. Androl..* 2010. 33:475–488. doi: 10.1111/j.1365-2605.2009.

Fischl., F., Riegler, R., Bieglmayer, C., et al. Modification of semen quality by acupuncture in subfertile males. *Geburtshilfe Frauenheilkd*. 1984. 44:510-512.

Gradini, R., Realacci, M., Petrangeli, E., et al. Nitric oxide synthases in normal and benign hyperplastic human prostate: immunohistochemistry and molecular biology. *J. Pathol.* 1999. 189: 224–229

Hsueh, T. Herb-Drug Interaction of Epimedium sagittatum (Sieb. Et. Zucc.) Maxim Extract on Pharmacokinetics of Sildenafil in Rats. *Molecules*. 2013. 18: 7323-7335.

Kho, H.G., Sweep, C.G., Chen, X., et al. The use of acupuncture in the treatment of erectile dysfunction. *Int. J. Impot. Res.* 1999. 11:41-46.

Kim, S. F. The role of nitric oxide in prostaglandin biology; update. *Nitric Oxide.* 2011. 25: 255–264. doi:10.1016/j.niox.2011.07.002

Klein, R., Klein, B.E.,Tomany, S.C., et al. The relation of retinal microvascular characteristics to age-related eye disease: the Beaver Dam eye study. *Am. J. Ophthalmol.* 2004. 137:435-444.

Kyprianou, N. Doxazosin and terazosin suppress prostate growth by inducing apoptosis: clinical significance. *J. Urol.* 2003. 169:1520-1525.

Lee, S.H. and Lee, B.C. Electroacupuncture relieves pain in men with chronic prostatitis/chronic pelvic pain syndrome: three-arm randomized trial. *Urology.* 2009. 73:1036–1041. doi: 10.1016/j.urology.2008.10.047.

Lee, S.W., Liong, M.L., Yuen, K.H., et al. Acupuncture versus sham acupuncture for chronic prostatitis/chronic pelvic pain. *Am. J. Med.* 2008. 121:79.e1–7.

Morelli, A., Filippi, S., Comeglio, P., et al. Acute vardenafil administration improves bladder oxygenation in spontaneously hypertensive rats. *J. Sex Med.* 2010. 7:107-120. doi: 10.1111/j.1743-6109.2009.01558.x.

Oelke, M., Bachmann, A., Descazeaud, A., et al. EAU guidelines on the treatment and follow-up of non-neurogenic male lower urinary tract symptoms including benign prostatic obstruction. *Eur. Urol.* 2013. 64:118-140. doi: 10.1016/j.eururo.2013.03.004.

Philp, T., Shah, P.J., and Worth, P.H. Acupuncture in the treatment of bladder instability. *Br. J. Urol.* 1988. 61: 490–493.

Ricci, L., Minardi, D., Romoli, M., et al. Acupuncture reflexotherapy in the treatment of sensory urgency that persists after transurethral resection of the prostate: a preliminary report. *Neurourol. Urodyn.* 2004. 23:58-62.

Rittmaster, R.S. 5alpha-reductase inhibitors in benign prostatic hyperplasia and prostate cancer risk reduction. *Best Pract. Res. Clin. Endocrinol. Metab.* 2008. 22:389-402. doi: 10.1016/j.beem.2008.01.016.

Sahin, S., Bicer, M., Eren, G.A., et al. Acupuncture relieves symptoms in chronic prostatitis/chronic pelvic pain syndrome: a randomized, sham-controlled trial. *Prostate Cancer Prostatic Dis.* 2015. 18:249–254. doi: 10.1038/pcan.2015.13.

Schröder, S., Liepert, J., Remppis, A., et al. Acupuncture treatment improves nerve conduction in peripheral neuropathy. *Eur. J. Neurol.* 2007. 14:276-281.

Shin, S.J., Lee, K.H., Chung, K.S., et al. The traditional Korean herbal medicine Ga-Gam-Nai-Go-Hyan suppresses testosterone-induced benign prostatic hyperplasia by regulating inflammatory responses and apoptosis. *Exp. Ther, Med.* 2017. 13:1025-1031. doi: 10.3892/etm.2017.4088.

Wang, Y., Liu, B., Yu, J., et al. Electroacupuncture for moderate and severe benign prostatic hyperplasia: a randomized controlled trial. *PLoS ONE.* 2013. 8:e59449. doi: 10.1371/journal.pone.0059449.

Wang, Y., Liu, Z., Yu, J., et al. Efficacy of electroacupuncture at Zhongliao point (BL33) for mild and moderate benign prostatic hyperplasia: study protocol for a randomized controlled trial. *Trials.* 2011. 12: 211. doi:10.1186/1745-6215-12-211.

Zheng, R., and Hu, H. Impacts of electroacupuncture on benign prostatic hyperplasia and the levels of estrogen and androgen in patients. *Zhongguo Zhen Jiu.* 2017. 37:599-602. doi: 10.13703/j.0255-2930.2017.06.007.

Zhou, J. Icariin and its derivative, ICT, exert anti-inflammatory, antitumor effects, and modulate myeloid derived suppressive cells (MDSCs) functions. *Int. Immunopharmacol.* 2011. 11: 887-895.

INDEX

www.ingramcontent.com/pod-product-compliance
Lightning Source LLC
Chambersburg PA
CBHW070759260726
48660CB00005B/1686